Sharira Unveiled:

The Body's Forgotten Secrets

Ancient Wisdom Meets Modern Health

Ancient Roots,

Timeless Well-being,

Modern Relevance.

Published by Guru Educircle Publications, Mumbai, India.
support@gurueducircle.com

First Edition: August 2025

ISBN: 978-81-993219-9-1 Printed in India.

Design and Layout by **Hojayega. Creative house**

Cover Illustration by **Rucha Bajaj.**

Disclaimers

Your journey to radiant health is sacred, and *Sharira Unveiled* is your guide to nurturing your body's wisdom. This book is intended for informational and educational purposes only and is not a substitute for professional medical advice, diagnosis, or treatment. The content, including advice on Ayurveda, yoga, mindfulness, diet, exercise, and lifestyle practices, is based on the author's personal experiences, traditional wisdom, and general research, and should not be considered a medical recommendation.

Before adopting the practices described, please consult a qualified healthcare provider or a Sukh-Arogyam expert (reachable at support@sukharogyam.com or www.sukharogyam.com). Individual results may vary, and certain practices may not be suitable for everyone, especially those with pre-existing medical conditions, pregnant or nursing individuals, or those on medication.

The author, Dr. Tanmay Jaju, and Guru Educircle Publications disclaim any liability for any loss, injury, or damage incurred by readers as a result of using or relying upon the information contained herein. The inclusion of quotes, data, or references does not imply endorsement by those sources, and permissions or licenses (where applicable) are noted in the References section. Let *Sharira Unveiled* be your first step toward a vibrant, balanced life. Begin with care and wisdom under professional guidance.

To my family and the timeless wisdom of our ancestors, may this journey inspire us all to weave health, happiness, and soul into every thread of our lives.

Sukh-Arogyam

/sukh-a·rog·yam/

Sukh

/sukh/

1. a state of inner joy, contentment, and ease not dependent on external circumstances but within.
2. Derived from the Sanskrit root "su" (good) + "kha" (space or axle), originally meaning "a smooth-running chariot," symbolizing a smooth flow of life.
3. The felt sense of harmony comes when one is in tune with the truth and nature.

Arogyam

/a·rog·yam/

1. Complete health and well-being, a dynamic equilibrium of the body, mind, emotions, and spirit.
2. from the Sanskrit root "a" (absence) + "roga" (disease or dis-ease), meaning "freedom from disease."
3. not merely the absence of illness, but the presence of vitality, clarity, strength, and serenity

Contents

Introduction

Sukh-Arogyam to all.

We live in an age that measures achievement but forgets the vessel that holds it. Sharira Unveiled is a short, practical companion for anyone who wants to reverse that forgetting. At its heart is one proposition: Sukh-Arogyam (true well-being) is not merely the absence of disease but the harmonious unfolding of seven interdependent petals, Sharira (body), Manas (mind), Bhava (emotions), Sambandh (relationships), Dhan (resources), Paryavaran (environment), and Atma (soul). When one petal wilts, the whole lotus fades; when one is tended, all bloom.

This book is structured to be lived, not just read. Each chapter homes in on a petal or principle: the body as temple, the inner code of Prakriti, the mechanics of Prana and Agni, the origins of imbalance, and practical pathways back to rhythm. Expect concise theory, concrete daily practices (dinacharya), brief reflections, and a simple inquiry practice I call Anusandhan , a one-page mirror for honest self-awareness.

If you are pressed for time, use the "One Mirror" and the short action plans at the end of each chapter. If you are searching for depth, read the stories and reflective prompts. Above all, treat this book as an invitation: not to perform perfectly, but to remember the life already seeded within you. Begin here, with a small breath. The rest follows.

Preface

"A Doctor's Vow to Your Sacred Sharira"

The benediction at my wedding still sounds in my ears: "शतायुर्भव, may you live a hundred years." It was spoken with the same tenderness my elders have always offered, and yet that night my wife and I laughed and asked, almost defiantly, "Is that even possible?" The question stayed with me. Over the years, it returned in small scenes, a brilliant student working through midnight oil until his health faltered, a teacher who preserved breath and body into old age, a friend startled by the vitality of a 97-year-old executive who insisted on driving himself. These moments were not statistics; they were knocks at the door of a deeper truth: longevity and joy are not accidents of fate but crafts we can learn.

I write this book from the seat of that curiosity, as a practitioner, a son of daily rituals, and a student of both ancient texts and modern science. My work with people taught me that crises rarely begin as catastrophes. They begin as small betrayals of the body: missed meals, erased sleep, rushed breath. They ripple outward and dim everything we care for. Yet I have also seen how a single, steady practice, an evening of presence, a mindful meal, a breath taken with intention, can reverse that slide.

Sharira Unveiled is my attempt to return us to our first temple: the body. It is a compassionate, practical map, part story, part ritual, part clinical observation, born of lived encounters and long study. If you take one thing from these pages, let it be this: care for the vessel, and everything you love will have a better chance to flourish.

Dr. Tanmay Jaju

Mumbai, 2025

Sharira Unveiled:

The Body's Forgotten Secrets

Ancient Wisdom Meets Modern Health

Chapter 1:
The Lotus of Wholeness

"देहं देवालयं प्रोक्तं जीवो देवः सनातनः।"

Deham devalayam proktam jivo devah sanatanah.

The body is said to be a temple; the soul is the eternal deity.

The Silent War: A Moment of Disconnect

Sukh-Arogyam to all my brothers and sisters.

It is a greeting. A blessing. A path.

It means

May you live a blissful, vibrant, and complete life, with radiant health and joyful harmony flowing through every dimension of your being.

"In seeking happiness, we often walk away from it." – Ancient proverb.

What if the life you're chasing is the one you're destroying? We are travellers in a restless world, as if running into a storm we created. We trade sleep for deadlines, our laughter for ambition, and with a presence for the hollow promise of "someday." We tell ourselves all lies to keep going:

> *"This is just temporary."*

> *"This is what everyone does."*

> *"This is how success feels, right?"*

Picture a family dinner, once alive with stories, now silenced by screens glowing in tired hands. This is not rare. It is the heartbeat of our new ordinary.

If you pause and notice, you'll see how casually we give away our laughter, always wagering on a tomorrow that often never comes. We starve today's joy, convinced we'll feast on happiness later, only to find the table cleared, the moment gone.

This isn't just a mistake; it's a betrayal of our own hearts. It's a silent war raging within us, where we sabotage the very wholeness we crave. We live the cruelest paradox: striving for a vibrant, complete life while unraveling the threads of our own well-being. But hear me out:

You are not broken; you are simply out of rhythm.

Imagine a musician, smashing the strings of his beloved instrument, convinced that silence will give him the perfect song.

Madness?

Yet don't we do the same? Fighting harder against our own well-being, burning the very vessel meant to bring us joy and peace. We push our limits, hurting our body, mind, emotions, and soul, the instruments of our happy life. We smash it and uproot it, and believe we'll earn peace and well-being at the end of it all.

But how can peace bloom in soil soaked with neglect? How can joy arrive in a home where we've evicted our own breath? This paradox is not just ours. It has echoed across centuries. The story of Great Valmiki reminds us that misalignment is not new; it is human.

The Mirror of Valya: A Return to Wholeness

Centuries ago, a fierce dacoit named Valya Koli terrorized the forests. His life was built upon violence and fear, his days spent ambushing travelers. His motive? To provide prosperity, well-being, and happiness for his family. Every plunder, every threat, every act of violence, he believed, was for them. He believed he carried the weight of survival for all.

One day, Valya lunged from the shadows, blade drawn, ready to rob yet another traveler. But this time, his target was a sage, radiant and unmoved. The sage looked him calmly in the eye and asked, "Why do this, even when you know this is wrong?"

"For my family," Valya replied, without hesitation.

"And will they share the consequences of your deeds?" the sage asked.

Valya scoffed. “Of course! Everything I do is for them!”

The sage gently said, “Go and ask them. I will stay here.”

Valya, confident and certain of their loyalty, went home and asked his mother, father, wife, and even his children, each one of them, more or less, had the same answer: "We all love you, but we eat what you bring. Your **karma** (कर्म, deeds/consequences), your deeds, are yours alone. Any consequence from it is your own."

Shattered, Valya returned.

The realignment...

The sage, full of compassion, offered a path: "Sit. Chant **Japa** (जप, meditative chanting). Let the name of the Divine reshape you."

Valya tried, but even the word "Rama" wouldn’t come. So, the sage reversed it: "Say 'Mara... Mara...'" (meaning 'dead'), which slowly softened into "Rama." Through years of unwavering meditation and profound inner purification, Valya transformed into the greatest sage, **Maharshi Valmiki**. This is the story of how Valya became Valmiki, the sage who composed the Ramayana, a testament to his inner revolution. Valmiki's story is our mirror. Like Valya, we justify our chaos for the sake of our loved ones, our perceived duties, and our future security. But the physical and emotional burdens we carry from our actions, from the choices we make for our bodies, are ours alone. No one else can bear them. This truth is not only sung in ancient scriptures. Even modern science, in its own language, now confirms what sages have always known.

A Global Crisis, A Timeless Path

This misalignment is not only Valmiki's story; it is ours. The world is paying the price for forgetting the body. Illness today often doesn't come from outside threats alone. It grows quietly out of how we live the way we eat, breathe, sleep, and move.

The World Health Organization warns of a silent wave: diabetes, heart disease, and exhaustion spreading faster than ever. In Japan, they even have a word for it, *Karoshi*, death by overwork. In America and Europe, depression and burnout rise like a tide no one can escape.

But these are not distant headlines. They are mirrors. Look at your own body: your sleep, your breath, your digestion. Where do you recognize yourself in these warnings? Where has your temple already begun to whisper for help?

What We Really Seek: A Living Temple

We crave peace, but cut short our rest.

We crave connection, but often scroll in silence.

We talk a lot about health, but treat our bodies as the last thing.

We dream of joy, but postpone it to one more goal.

But you are not a machine to be optimized.

You are a living temple.

This path is not about punishment or perfection. It is about remembrance, rhythm, and realignment. When you remember, you awaken. When you realign, life regains its rhythm. Together, they form the pulse of Sukh-Arogyam.

What is Sukh-Arogyam?

It is not a technique. It is a way of life.

- **Sukh (सुख) = Easeful joy, deep harmony, a state of profound Bliss.** This is the aspiration of a life lived with grace.
- **Arogyam (आरोग्यम्) = Radiant wellness, not merely the absence of disease, but a state of complete vitality, vibrant energy, and optimal functioning across every system of your being.**

This is the aspiration of a body in effortless flow.

Together: **Sukh-Arogyam (सुख-आरोग्यम्)**

When these two states unite, we rediscover a way of living that is frictionless, fluid, whole.

To live Sukh-Arogyam is to rise with lightness, eat with awareness, work with purpose, rest without guilt, and love without fear, not as tasks to tick off, but as a natural rhythm of being.

This is not about living in the past. It's about living like yourself, in present-time alignment with timeless truths.

"स्वस्थस्य स्वास्थ्य रक्षणं, आतुरस्य विकार प्रशमनं।"

(Swasthasya swasthya rakshanam, aturasya vikara prashamanam) – Charaka Samhita

Preserving the health of the healthy and treating the illness of the sick.

This is the call of Sukh-Arogyam: not to wait for disease, but to cultivate vitality in every breath, every step, every dimension of life.

The Seven Petals of Sukh-Arogyam: Your Lotus of Wholeness

Imagine your life as a beautiful lotus, its petals slowly opening up in morning light, each one vital, interconnected, and alive. When one petal wilts, the whole lotus dims. These are your seven petals of wholeness. They are complete aspects to make your life whole.

- **Sharira (शरीर – Body): The Sacred Vessel, blossomed.** This petal reflects your physical health, cellular vitality, breath, movement, and conscious nutrition. It's the primal architecture, the temple of **Prana** (प्राण), your life force.
- **Manas (मनस् – Mind): The Restless River, Calmed.** This petal holds your mental clarity, focus, cognition, memory, and thought flow. It's about a mind that serves rather than distracts.

- **Bhava (भाव – Emotions): The Inner Climate, Awakened.** This petal pulses with emotional intelligence, self-regulation, peace, joy, and compassion. It seeks emotional sovereignty.
- **Sambandh (सम्बन्ध – Relationships): The Golden Threads of Connection.** This petal embodies authentic bonds with family, friends, community, and humanity.
- **Dhan (धन – Wealth): The Fertile Soil of Abundance.** This petal goes beyond money, embracing sustainable abundance, wise choices, and joyful contribution.
- **Paryavaran (पर्यावरण – Environment): The Nurturing Breeze.** This petal links you to your ecological, digital, and spiritual surroundings.
- **Atma (आत्मा – Soul/Spirit): The Eternal Flame, Unveiled.** This petal reflects your **dharma** (धर्म), spiritual connection, Higher Self, and sacred purpose. It seeks a life of deep meaning, inner peace, and authentic expression.

Together, these seven petals form **Sukh-Arogyam**, a living, breathing wholeness that transcends metrics and achievements, radiating joy from every corner of your being.

The Interplay of the Petals: A Living Ecosystem

A lotus does not bloom in fragments.

No petal can shine while another withers.

This is the philosophy of **Sukh-Arogyam**:

Your body, mind, emotions, relationships, wealth, environment, and soul are not seven separate stories. They are one living ecosystem.

Think of a time you lost sleep for weeks. Did your mind stay sharp? Or did your thoughts grow foggy, your patience thin, your emotions raw? Perhaps even your relationships felt the strain.

Think of a season when you felt anxious or heavy-hearted. Did food taste the same? Did work flow with ease? Or did every task feel heavier, every joy muted?

Think of the times you were vibrant, well-rested, eating clean, breathing deeply. On those days, wasn't love easier, laughter freer, focus sharper, even your sense of purpose brighter?

This is the truth of your lotus:

- One petal distorted the whole Sukh-Arogyam collapses.
- One petal nourished lifts the other towards Sukh-Arogyam.

"सर्वं खल्विदं ब्रह्म।"

Sarvam khalvidam brahma. – Chandogya Upanishad

All this is indeed whole; everything is interconnected.

Sukh-Arogyam is not about fixing one piece at a time. It is about remembering that you are already whole. The petals rise and fall together. The bloom opens only when all are tended. **Sukh-Arogyam** is your beacon in this storm. It is an integrated path, blending Ayurveda's timeless insights with cutting-edge modern science, offering a profound, actionable way to reclaim your wholeness.

"असतो मा सद्गमय, तमसो मा ज्योतिर्गमय, मृत्योर्मा अमृतं गमय।"

Asato ma sadgamaya, tamaso ma jyotirgamaya, mrityorma amritamgamaya. – Brihadaranyaka Upanishad

Lead me from untruth to truth, from darkness to light, from death to immortality.

For Reflection

Do not rush these questions. Let them be with you for a while to make you feel the reflection. Read one, pause, breathe, and allow your body to answer before your mind does.

1. **The Weight You Carry:** The Valmiki story reminds us that our choices return to us alone. Where are you giving away your well-being, body, mind, or emotions, in the name of duty, love, or ambition? Notice how this sacrifice in one petal quietly pulls the others down with it.
2. **The Promise of 'Someday':** In the past week, where did you delay joy, rest, or connection, telling yourself you would return to it later? Did that postponement only touch one part of your life, or did it ripple across your energy, your patience, your bonds?
3. **The Voice of Your Petals:** Every petal speaks when it is strained. Your body may whisper through fatigue, your mind through fog, your emotions through heaviness. When was the last time one petal spoke and you ignored it? What cost did the others pay for that silence?
4. **The Petal That Waits:** Among the seven petals of Sukh-Arogyam, which feels open and nourished today? Which one feels fragile, waiting for your attention? What is one small, gentle act you can take this week to water that petal, so that the whole lotus may begin to bloom again?

A Call to Begin: The Dawn of Awareness

Anusandhan: The First Step

Every healing begins with seeing.

The first step to solving any problem is not rushing to fix it; it is to understand it.

Mindfulness itself is our first medicine.

When we notice what is out of rhythm, we are already halfway back to alignment.

This practice of awareness is called **Anusandhan**, a gentle inquiry, a mindful looking within.

So, where do we begin? With our petals.

How to Practice Anusandhan

1. **Take a notebook.** This will be your *Sukh-Arogyam Journal.*
2. **Choose one petal at a time.** Start with *Sharira* (Body).
3. **Write two lists:**
    - *Five things that trouble me in this petal.* (e.g., "I wake up tired," "I eat in a hurry," "My shoulders ache.")
    - *Five things that nourish me in this petal.* (e.g., "A walk in fresh air," "Eating warm food," "Stretching in the morning.")

4. **If you feel blank, don't worry.** We will offer guiding prompts in this book and through the Sukh-Arogyam app to help you reflect. Even noticing one thing is enough.

Do this not only for the body, but for each petal of your lotus:

- **Sharira (Body):** Where do I feel strain? Where do I feel strength?
- **Manas (Mind):** When does my mind serve me? When does it scatter me?
- **Bhava (Emotions):** What emotions uplift me? What emotions weigh me down?
- **Sambandh (Relationships):** Which bonds give me life? Which ones drain me?
- **Dhan (Wealth):** What choices feel abundant? What habits feel depleting?
- **Paryavaran (Environment):** What surroundings nourish me? What exhausts me?
- **Atma (Soul):** When do I feel close to my purpose? When do I feel lost?

Gentle Reminder

This is not an exam.

You are not here to judge yourself.

Even writing a single line for each petal is enough to begin.

Anusandhan is awareness, not perfection.

By seeing clearly, you have already watered the lotus of your life

beginning.

Toward the First Petal

You have now begun your Anusandhan, your gentle inquiry into the petals of your own lotus. By noticing what nourishes you and what strains you, you have already taken the first step toward Sukh-Arogyam.

Remember this truth: **no petal stands alone.** When one dims, the whole lotus feels its shadow. When one is nourished, the whole flower lifts.

But every lotus has a root. Every petal rests on a foundation.

That foundation is **Sharira, the body.**

It is the vessel of your Prana, the chariot for your soul, the ground from which every other petal draws its strength. Without Sharira, no other petal can fully bloom.

In the next chapter, we begin here, with the body as your first temple.

We will rediscover why the ancients revered Sharira as the base of dharma, and how honoring it is the beginning of all wholeness.

Let us walk into the first petal of Sukh-Arogyam. Let us return to Sharira.

Chapter 2:
Sharira: The Sacred Foundation

"नायमात्मा बलहीनेन लभ्यः"

Nayamatma balahinena labhyah – Mundaka Upanishad

The Self is not attained by the weak body and will.

A Whisper Before the First Note

In Chapter 1, we faced the silent ache of our time, the cost of chasing happiness without wholeness. We explored **Sukh-Arogyam** (the harmonious union of easeful joy and radiant wellness), a forgotten melody of easeful joy and vitality.

But where do we begin to reclaim this lost harmony?

Imagine a flute trying to be played without breath, or a house with cracked foundations. In the same way, a neglected body cannot sustain itself in true well-being. The first note of your life's music is **Sharira**, if we consider the body as our musical instrument...

The *Rigveda* whispers a timeless truth:

"शरीरं यदवाप्नोति यच्च तेजः संहितम्।"

"Shariram yad avapnoti yachcha tejah"—Rigveda

"The body is the vessel that holds your divine light."

The Blessed Flame: Ramanujan and the Forgotten Temple

In the early 1900s, a young man named Srinivasa Ramanujan sat alone in a small house in South India, scribbling equations on scraps of paper. To him, mathematics was not arithmetic; it was revelation. He said that every formula was shown to him by the goddess Namagiri. His notebooks were filled not with calculations, but with visions, fragments of the infinite.

By his thirties, without formal training, he had touched realms of knowledge that the world's greatest mathematicians had not yet imagined. He was a flame of genius, a mind lit by the divine.

But the same flame that lit his mind consumed his body. In his devotion to numbers, he forgot the vessel that carried him. His meals were irregular, his rest broken, his Sharira, his temple, was neglected. His body grew frail, and at the age of just 32, the flame went out.

What might humanity have gained if Ramanujan had lived a hundred years? What worlds of science would he have revealed if he had tended the body that housed his soul? His equations remain with us, but the centuries of wisdom he could have given were lost to neglect.

Now, place beside him another son of India: T. Krishnamacharya, born in the same era. He, too, was blessed, not with numbers, but with breath, movement, and discipline. He honored his Sharira. He nourished his body, tended his Prana, and aligned with nature's rhythm. He lived to nearly a hundred, carrying vitality to his last days.

And because he lived, he gave. He revived yoga, trained disciples who carried it across the world, B.K.S. Iyengar, Pattabhi Jois, and Indra Devi. Through him, millions found strength, health, and balance. His legacy continues to breathe in countless bodies even today.

Two lives, two legacies. Both were touched by greatness, yet one ended too soon while the other flourished for decades. The message is simple: talent alone is not enough; the body must endure for the gift to last.

Without Sharira, brilliance fades. With Sharira, even ordinary effort can echo across centuries.

And the same truth is alive in our own time. Roger Federer, the maestro of tennis, played into his late thirties with a grace that seemed almost effortless. His longevity was not luck. It was discipline, recovery, and respect for his Sharira. By listening to his body, he extended not only his career but the joy he gave to millions.

What is Sharira?

At its most fundamental, Sharira is your body, the vessel through which you live and experience the world. It is breath and blood, strength and sensation, the rhythm of your days and nights. But in the vision of Sukh-Arogyam, Sharira is more than biology. It is your living temple, the sacred ground that holds your consciousness, carries your Prana (life energy), and serves as the first instrument of your actions and your spiritual journey.

"शरीरमाद्यं खलु धर्मसाधनम्।"

Shariramadyam khalu dharma sadhanam. – Charaka Samhita,

The body is the first instrument of dharma, the foundation for purpose, for righteous action, for the way your life serves truth.

This is not new wisdom. Our ancestors revered Sharira as a divine temple. They rose with the sun's rhythm, ate with the seasons, and moved with the grace of the Earth. Their bodies were not burdens; they were chariots for the soul, vessels where joy, purpose, and divinity intertwined.

The Body: A Temple Then, a Battleground Now, and a Beacon If We Act

In 2014, I stood beside my bride under the sacred canopy of Indian tradition. The air carried the scent of sandalwood, and the chants echoed blessings of eternity. As we bowed to our elders, most of them placed their hands over our heads and uttered the timeless benediction:

"शतायुर्भव" – *Shatayurbhava* – May you live a hundred years.

Later that evening, my wife and I laughed softly. "*Is this even possible?*" we wondered. Most people begin to wither by 60. By 70, many are gone. If 80 is reached, it is often with frailty, illness, and dependence. Where did those hundred years go? This is not just our story. It is a shared global reality.

There was a time when the body, Sharira, was revered as a sanctum. People rose with the sun, ate with the seasons, honored rest, and moved in harmony with the Earth. Their bodies were not just healthy; they were alive with rhythm.

But somewhere, we traded that temple for a touchscreen. Today, our nights glow with screens instead of moonlight. We move less, breathe shallow, and often eat food stripped of its roots. We guard our phones with software, yet leave our own bodies unprotected against stress, restlessness, and exhaustion.

We know more than any generation before us, yet our bodies carry more inflammation and fatigue than ever. We are more connected online, yet more disconnected from the very body that carries our soul.

The real tragedy isn't death itself, but the slow decline we accept while still living. This is not defeat by disease, but by daily neglect. A temple needs tending. A fire needs fuel. A soul needs a body to serve, to rise, to fulfill dharma.

We did not lose ancient wisdom. We stopped listening. We fell asleep in comfort, mistaking convenience for progress. But life always calls us back, sometimes as a whisper, sometimes as a storm, reminding us that the body must once again become our first temple.

Echoes Across Time: The Body's Role in Greatness

History whispers a truth through every generation: without the body, brilliance dims.

Now imagine this man. For over two decades, he moved across courts like flowing poetry, every stroke an expression of grace, every match a masterclass in composure. He won **20 Grand Slam titles**, held the World No. 1 ranking for **310 weeks**, and even as his hair turned silver at the edges, he was still lifting trophies against men ten years younger.

Fans do speak of him not just as an athlete, but as an artist. Watching him play often felt like watching poetry in motion.

He was admired not only for how much he won, but for how long he stayed at the top. His greatness was not a brief spark; it was a steady flame that burned across decades.

Who is he?

Roger Federer. A legend not only of tennis, but of longevity.

And here lies the secret: his genius was not only in his talent, but in his care. Federer respected his Sharira. He trained, yes, but he also recovered. He worked, but he also rested. He honored rhythm, discipline, and renewal as much as skill. He treated his body not as a machine to be exploited, but as a temple to be tended.

This is why he endured. This is why his career stretched into years that most athletes never reach. And this is why his story is more than sport; it is proof of a timeless truth:

Legends are created not only by brilliance, but by longevity. And longevity is born from protecting your Sharira first.

Without Sharira, brilliance fades too soon. With Sharira, even ordinary effort becomes extraordinary, and genius becomes legacy.

Sharira: The Launchpad for Every Petal's Bloom

Your Sharira is more than a body; it is the launchpad for every petal's journey. Consider its power: a rested Sharira steadies Atma (the soul) for meditation, its vitality fuelling spiritual ascent. A nourished Sharira strengthens Dhan (wealth), where productivity turns into prosperity. Research shows that healthy employees are nearly 20% more effective. A strong Sharira deepens Sambandh (relationships), giving the energy to connect, while a neglected body breeds distance and fatigue.

Modern science agrees. *The Lancet* reminds us that consistent movement can extend life by nearly 40%, yet we still sit, scroll, and sacrifice. Sharira demands attention, now, in youth to build resilience, in stress to restore balance, and always in daily life, whether at your desk, in a garden, or in prayer.

Actionable Engagement:

Take a moment now. Notice your breath. Is it shallow or deep? Consciously lengthen it for three slow counts. This small act is already your first offering to Sharira.

The Chariot, The King, and The Eternal Journey

Picture this: Your soul is a king, wise and noble, yearning to fulfill its **Dharma**. **Sharira** is the chariot, sturdy and true, carrying the king toward destiny. The senses are the horses, eager to run, and the mind the reins, guiding the course. Without a sound chariot, the journey falters, no matter the king's vision or the horses' strength.

The Bhagavad Gita advises,

शरीरं यदवाप्नोति यच्चाप्युत्क्रामतीश्वरः।

Shariram yad avapnoti yac capy utkramatisvarah

The soul enters and leaves through the body." Honor it, and the path opens.

Gandhi knew: "It is health that is real wealth and not pieces of gold and silver."

Every wisdom tradition points to the same truth: **Sharira is the container of the cosmos. Treat it as a footnote, and the chariot cracks. Tend it as your first temple, and it becomes your beacon.**

A vibrant Sharira brings boundless energy, sharp focus, emotional steadiness, social vitality, and spiritual receptivity. A weak Sharira invites fatigue, fog, irritability, and missed opportunities. The choice is yours. The question is not *if* Sharira matters, but *when* you will choose to honor it.

The Domino Effect: Whispers to Warnings

When Sharira begins to falter, the decline is rarely isolated. One wheel slips, and the whole procession feels the strain.

A whisper of stiffness, a little fatigue, these are signals of a loose wheel. Ignore them, and the wobble spreads: the mind loses clarity (Manas), emotions sour (Bhava), relationships fray (Sambandh). Push further, and the chariot halts, dimming prosperity (Dhan) and even spirit (Atma).

This is the domino effect: one petal weakened, and the whole lotus dims.

For Reflection

Do not rush these questions. Let them sit with you like a friend at help. Read one, pause, breathe, and allow your body to answer before your mind does.

1. **The Chariot's Cry:** Where is your body sending you a quiet signal, fatigue, stiffness, pain, that you have been ignoring? If you continue to neglect it, how might that one wheel begin to shake the whole chariot of your life?
2. **The Short Flame vs. The Steady Flame:** Ramanujan's brilliance was cut short by neglect, while Krishnamacharya's care gave him a century of impact. Which flame are you living right now, burning fast, or burning steady?
3. **The Secret of Longevity:** Federer's greatness was not only in his victories but in his endurance. What one practice could you bring into your daily rhythm, rest, movement, recovery, that would help you extend your own legacy?
4. **Beyond the Surface:** Your Sharira is not only a tool for work, but the temple of your dharma. Sit with your breath. Ask yourself: *What deeper purpose does my body serve? What does it need from me to carry that purpose with strength?*

Action Plan: The One Mirror of Sharira

If Chapter 1 opened your eyes to the seven petals, then Chapter 2 brings you to the root, the Sharira. This step is not casual. It may be the most important practice of this book.

Most people fail here. They ignore their body until pain forces attention, until illness steals choice, until it feels too late. Do not wait for a crisis. If you can win this one practice, truly honoring and listening to your Sharira, then every other change will feel lighter, easier, and natural.

This is not repetition. This is the foundation. Without it, no practice will hold. With it, every practice will flow.

The One Mirror Practice

Take a quiet moment. Sit comfortably. Place one hand on your chest, the other on your stomach. Close your eyes. Let your breath settle.

Now ask your body three questions:

1. **What gives me strength?** (What in my body feels alive, steady, or resilient?)
2. **What feels strained?** (Where do I sense weakness, discomfort, or neglect?)
3. **What is my body asking for today?** (Rest, movement, nourishment, touch, stillness?)

Write **just three lines** in your Sukh-Arogyam Journal:

- One strength.
- One strain.
- One request.

That is enough.

Why This Matters

This is not a daily task. You do this once, and already the mirror is clear. Even a single honest entry will plant a seed of awareness that begins to grow on its own.

If you avoid this step, the path ahead will feel like effort, like pushing against yourself. If you take this step, the path will feel like alignment, because you will be walking with your Sharira, not against it.

This is why Sharira-Vimarsha, the One Mirror practice, is the true starting point of this journey.

If you want, you can track these reflections on the **Sukh-Arogyam app**, where gentle reminders and guiding prompts will help you notice how your strengths grow, how your strains ease, and how your body's requests change over time.

Do not underestimate this practice. Many people fail here because it looks simple. But those who win here unlock the door to everything else,

Toward the Next Chapter: Sharira Through the Lens of Sukh-Arogyam

You have now seen Sharira as your first temple, the vessel that carries your dharma, the launchpad for every petal of your lotus. In this chapter, you held a mirror to your body, listening to its strengths, its strains, and its deepest requests. That one act of seeing may already have shifted something inside you.

But Sharira does not exist alone. It is not a separate island. Every breath, every ache, every surge of energy ripples outward, into your mind, your emotions, your relationships, your prosperity, your environment, your very soul.

This is where the philosophy of Sukh-Arogyam becomes your compass. It teaches us that Sharira is not just one petal among seven; it is the ground from which the whole lotus draws life. To understand your body through the Sukh-Arogyam lens is to see how its whispers are connected to every corner of your being.

In the next chapter, we step into that lens. We will explore how Sharira speaks to you, not in words, but in signals: discomforts, imbalances, and quiet aches that are not enemies but guides. These are not punishments. They are the body's way of calling you back into rhythm.

Sharira is not just your foundation. It is your messenger. in learning and listening to it is the key to living whole.

Chapter 3:

Beyond the Machine: Your Body's Ancient Blueprint

"धन्यं स्वास्थ्यं परं सुखम्।"

Dhanyam svasthyam param sukham.-sushruta samhita

"Health is the greatest wealth, supreme happiness."

A Luminous Life, not a Quiet Decline

In Chapter 2, we awakened to a profound truth: your Sharira, the physical body, is not a cage for your soul but a sacred chariot for your purpose. The legacies of the great minds and sages were not built on relentless striving, but on the disciplined care of their bodies.

But if the body is a temple, how do we learn its language? How do we read its intricate story, not as a list of symptoms, but as a path back to wholeness?

Today, we risk forgetting. We have reduced this sacred vessel to a collection of parts, a machine to be optimized. We say, "*I'm running on coffee and stress*," as if our bodies were fuel tanks. We chase easy rewards in dopamine while ignoring the quiet signals of fatigue. We spend a lot on supplements, while the cheapest, simplest, and most fundamental gifts, wholesome food, deep sleep, and natural movement, are mostly neglected.

This is not just a contradiction. It is a tragedy.

We are not designed for falling apart at sixty or resigning at eighty. The human body is created for full longevity, for a century of vitality, learning, giving, and joy. When someone dies in their early eighties and we call it "a full life," this shows how much we've lowered our expectations.

Your design is richer than quiet decline. You were meant not just to survive, but to move in rhythm with life, growing, giving, and thriving.

Driving at 97: A Life Rewritten

And yet, while some lives are cut short despite surface fitness, others shine well into the tenth decade. What makes the difference?

This vibrant longevity isn't a statistical anomaly; it's the remarkable fruit of a holistic understanding; a life lived through the integrated wisdom we've begun exploring. It is a testament to what's possible when we truly honor our **Sharira**.

One evening last week, my dear friend Saurabh, a man of profound insight, shared an encounter that fundamentally reshaped his definition of aging.

He had embarked on a trip to Japan for a high-stakes business meeting with a client. They had only ever communicated through emails, so this was their first in-person encounter. After Saurabh completed his airport formalities, he walked out and instinctively scanned the crowd. He was expecting a young executive, perhaps a uniformed chauffeur holding a sign, but instead, a distinguished, almost impossibly spry 97-year-old man emerged, radiating a serene, vibrant energy. The owner of the client company had come to pick him up himself. He stood by a new black Lexus, smiling warmly, his eyes holding a depth of wisdom that transcended his immaculate suit.

As they moved toward the car, a wave of shock washed over Saurabh. He offered politely, "Sir, let me drive. I insist." He was taken aback not just by the man's age, but by his evident vitality and self-sufficiency.

The man chuckled, a deep, resonant sound that carried the wisdom of decades. His eyes twinkled with a delightful mischief. "Drive? My friend," he said softly, his voice clear and steady, "I didn't buy this car for you. I bought it for myself."

With that, he gracefully slid into the driver's seat, motioned Saurabh into the passenger seat, and expertly, confidently, navigated them through the bustling city traffic.

That day, for Saurabh, wasn't just a business meeting; it was a profound personal awakening. His ingrained definitions of aging and what was possible in life were utterly shattered. Here was a man thriving, engaging with the world, driving himself, working, dreaming, and living with undeniable zest at 97.

And here so many of us are, feeling the limitations of age by forty, worn out by fifty, and resigned to a quiet decline by sixty. This stark contrast needs our urgent attention, just think.

You were never meant to merely exist or to collapse prematurely. You were profoundly designed to carry light, wisdom, and vibrant energy for a century and beyond. This is your inherent birthright.

And yet, while some thrive into their tenth decade, others falter far too soon.

The Flawed Machine: A One-Dimensional View

Our modern approach to health is a testament to this flawed mindset. We treat the body as a machine, believing that if we just find the right fuel or the right upgrade, it will run forever. But life tells a more complex story.

We may fill our plates with superfoods, yet still feel incomplete. We may dedicate ourselves to disciplined fitness, yet remain vulnerable. The world has seen beloved figures, celebrated chefs, and admired actors who outwardly embodied health and vitality, yet were taken from us far too early.

Their stories are not failures of food or of fitness. They are reminders that true wellness cannot be reduced to diet or exercise alone. Health is not guaranteed by trends or routines; it demands a deeper listening, a fuller integration.

The truth is clear: we are not machines. We are intricate, interconnected systems of body, mind, and spirit. When we focus on only one part, the entire system remains fragile. The path of Sukh-Arogyam, the harmonious union of easeful joy and radiant wellness, is about moving beyond this narrow view, into a holistic picture of thriving.

The Sukh-Arogyam Kaleidoscope: Three Lenses to See Your Body

To truly understand what your body is whispering, you cannot look with a single, narrow lens. You must have something like a kaleidoscope, with three lenses, each revealing a different aspect of truth.

- One shows you the *why*.
- One shows you *how*.
- One shows you *what now*.

Together, they give you not fragments, but a whole.

Lens 1: Ancient Indian Wisdom — The Why

This is the philosophical foundation. It shows your body as a microcosm of the cosmos, composed of the Pancha Mahabhuta, the five great elements.

Akasha (Space) gives you room to exist.

Vayu (Air) brings movement and breath.

Agni (Fire) fuels transformation and energy.

Jala (Water) offers flow and cohesion.

Prithvi (Earth) gives structure and stability.

Your bones are Earth. Your blood is Water. Your digestion is Fire. Your breath is Air. The space between your cells is Akasha.

Your unique balance of these elements is not random; it is your nature, your rhythm, your dharma.

As within the body, so in the cosmos.

Lens 2: Ayurvedic Intelligence — The How

This is the practical instruction manual. Ayurveda teaches that your body is governed by three doshas, Vata, Pitta, and Kapha, the subtle forces that shape every function of body and mind.

It tells you to tend your Agni, the digestive fire that sustains life. When Agni weakens, Ama (toxins) spreads, and imbalance begins.

This lens gives you a personal roadmap: how to eat, how to move, how to rest, so that you stay aligned with your own elemental design.

When Agni burns steadily, balance flows steadily.

Lens 3: Modern Empowerment — The What Now

This is the bridge to today's world. It translates ancient truths into modern science.

It shows how chronic stress raises cortisol, how breath calms the nervous system, how movement reshapes the brain through neuroplasticity, and how community protects both immunity and longevity.

This lens is not separate from the ancient; it confirms it, in a language our times can understand.

Your biology is ancient wisdom written in modern code.

Together

These three lenses do not contradict. They complete one another. Turn them together, and the body is no longer a machine of parts but a living symphony. Through this kaleidoscope, you see the whole: a roadmap for thriving in harmony, across time and self.

The Ripple Beneath the Surface: A Holistic Glimpse

These three lenses, when viewed through the Sukh-Arogyam kaleidoscope, reveal Sharira's profound interconnectedness with every other petal of your being.

Take a common symptom: **chronic stress.**

- **Ancient Lens:** Stress is seen as a Vata (air and space) disturbance, disrupting the subtle flow of Prana (life force) and creating inner turbulence.
- **Ayurvedic Lens:** Stress weakens Agni (digestive fire), leading to the buildup of Ama (toxins) across the tissues (dhatus) and disturbing all three Doshas.
- **Modern Lens:** Stress appears as surges of cortisol, shallow breathing, and adrenal fatigue, biological proof of its toll on both mind and body.

Seen through these three lenses, stress stops looking like a small surface issue. It shows up as a thread woven through the whole of life.

- It clouds your **Manas** (mind), creating fog and anxiety.
- It sours your **Bhava** (emotions), manifesting as irritability and exhaustion.
- It strains your **Sambandh** (relationships), fraying bonds with those you love.
- It weakens your **Dhan** (financial well-being), lowering productivity and raising hidden costs.
- And at its deepest, it dims your **Atma** (soul), pulling you away from your sense of purpose.

For the professional under relentless deadlines, this might show up as back pain that no physiotherapy can fully explain. For the caregiver in an overburdened hospital, it might be exhaustion that no amount of sleep truly repairs.

These are not isolated complaints. They are messages, whispers from Sharira, reminding us to realign the entire lotus of our being.

For Reflection

1. **The Flawed Machine:** The stories of the superfood chef and the actor highlight that a narrow focus on diet or exercise alone is not enough for true wellness. In your own life, what part of your well-being have you been trying to "optimize" as if it were a machine, while neglecting other vital parts of your system?
2. **The Kaleidoscope View:** Think about a current health issue or a feeling of being unwell (e.g., persistent fatigue, a nagging ache, mental fog). Use the three lenses, Ancient, Ayurvedic, and Modern, to describe this issue. How does seeing it through all three lenses change your perspective on its cause and potential solution?
3. **The Age of Limitation:** The story of the 97-year-old Japanese man challenges our modern assumptions about aging. What are the limiting beliefs you hold about your own body's potential as you get older? How might these beliefs be impacting your health and choices right now?
4. **A Life Rewritten:** What small, daily habit or choice can you make today that embodies the kind of vibrant, engaged life you want to be living at 97? Think beyond a single action. What is a daily rhythm you can start to cultivate to rewrite your own story?

Action Plan: Ahara, Honoring What Enters Your Temple

If Sharira is your first temple, then food is its daily offering. What you place into your body is not just fuel, it is **Prana made visible**, the very substance from which your tissues, your thoughts, your emotions, and even your joy are woven.

The sages remind us:

"अन्नं न निन्द्यात् तद्व्रतम्। प्राणोऽन्नम्।"
Annam na nindyat, tad vratam. Prano 'nnam. – Taittiriya Upanishad
Food must never be disrespected; it is the vow. For food is life itself.

Ahara as Nourishment for All Petals

Food is not only for your stomach. It is not only for your muscles. It is not only for your mind. True Ahara nourishes *every petal of your lotus*:

- It strengthens your **Sharira** (body), building vitality.
- It clears your **Manas** (mind), sharpening clarity.
- It soothes your **Bhava** (emotions), creating balance and calm.

- It binds your **Sambandh** (relationships), for food shared is love multiplied.
- It shapes your **Dhan** (wealth), because health sustains your ability to create and prosper.
- It respects your **Paryavaran** (environment), for natural, seasonal eating aligns you with Earth's rhythm.
- And it fuels your **Atma** (soul), because food taken with reverence becomes prayer.

Eating carelessly doesn't just leave the body wanting; it leaves the whole self-undernourished. Eating with awareness feeds every part of you.

The Three Pillars of Ahara

The seers of Ayurveda gave timeless guidance on how to honor food through **quality, quantity, and time**.

1. Quality (Guna):

Eat what is natural, seasonal, and fresh. Food should be *samskar-yukta*, prepared with the right process, no more, no less. Avoid the extremes: not over-refined, not over-spiced, not overly sweet or salty. Strive for meals that balance the **shad-rasa**, the six tastes of Ayurveda (sweet, sour, salty, bitter, pungent, astringent), so your being feels complete.

Packaged and ultra-processed foods only mimic nourishment. Respect yourself enough and keep them at bay.

2. Quantity (Matra):

Sage Vagbhata offers simple but profound wisdom: divide your stomach into four parts,

- Two parts for solid food,
- One part for liquid,
- One part left empty for air and movement.

Yet today, we fill to the throat, and then wonder why disease comes calling. True nourishment is balance, not excess.

3. Time (Kala):

Never skip meals out of carelessness, nor eat when hunger is absent. For the healthy, eating without hunger is as harmful as suppressing hunger. For the unwell, healing begins by gently kindling or calming hunger as needed.

Remember: **too much, too little, or mistimed eating is a sin against your temple.**

A Note for the Modern Reader

In today's world of endless diet fads and advice, Sukh-Arogyam does not teach a one-size-fits-all prescription. Ahara must be aligned with your prakriti (constitution), your age, your season of life, and your current state of balance or imbalance. For every disease, Ayurveda prescribes a unique path of nourishment to restore harmony.

Still, some truths are universal:

- **Hydrate wisely:** Water is life. Sip warm or room-temperature water throughout the day; avoid extremes of ice-cold or over-sweetened drinks.
- **Avoid ultra-processed foods:** If it comes in a packet engineered for "taste," it is not food, it is interference.
- **Eat with attention:** Sit, slow down, chew well. Do not eat with screens or distractions. Let eating itself be meditation. s
- **Honor variety:** Include all six tastes (shaḍ-rasa) so the body feels satisfied and whole.
- **Respect individuality:** A diet that heals one may harm another. The path is personal; your Sukh-Arogyam app and resources can help you discover what suits your prakriti and present needs.

A Prayer Before Food

Food is not merely a substance; it is a blessing. Let every meal begin with gratitude:

"ॐ सह नाववतु। सह नौ भुनक्तु।"
Om saha navavatu, saha nau bhunaktu.
May we be protected together; may we be nourished together.

This remembrance transforms eating from habit into ritual, from consumption into communion.

In this way, Ahara becomes the **first conscious practice of Sukh-Arogyam**. Not a diet. Not a fad. An honoring.

What enters your temple shapes what flows through every petal of your being, body, mind, heart, relationships, prosperity, environment, and soul.

A Closing Note: The Body as Symphony, Not Burden

Sukh-Arogyam is not a rigid protocol or a fleeting health hack. It is the profound art of remembering that **Sharira** is your first sacred song, a magnificent instrument not to be constantly optimized or forced, but to be deeply honored, intimately understood, and harmoniously played. Your body is not in the way of your dream. It is the way.

Your Sharira is not a machine to be optimized or a problem to be silenced. It is more like music; if you listen closely, it can bring you back to yourself.

Next, we journey deeper, beyond these general principles and into the utterly unique blueprint of your own being. It's time to truly meet your **Prakriti** (your original, unique constitution), your original design, the elemental DNA of your **Doshas**, the intrinsic rhythm of your inner music. Because the body isn't one size fits all.

Next, we'll look at your Prakriti: the unique rhythm you were born with. In knowing it, you begin to live in your truest and strongest way.

Chapter 4:
Your Inner Code: Unlocking the Wisdom of Prakriti

"यः शरीरं सम्यगुपासते स देवताः तस्य अन्तः प्रकाशयन्ति।"

Yah śariram samyag-upasate, sa devatah tasya antah prakaśayanti.

One who honors and tends to the body with reverence, the inner divinity illuminates that being from within.

Your Universe Within

Why do two children, raised the same, taught the same, grow into such different bodies, minds, and hearts? The answer lies in your Prakriti, the body's sacred geometry. In Chapter 3, we explored Sharira, the physical body, as a sacred vessel, a living reflection of the cosmos. The Pancha Mahabhuta (five great elements: Space, Air, Fire, Water, Earth) compose every particle of our being. This truth invites us to see the body not as a machine, but as a microcosm of the universe.

Now, let us draw closer to the unique rhythm within you. Your Prakriti is that rhythm, your original design, your inner code. It is the blueprint of your vitality, resilience, and a kind of inner guide to how you move through life. To understand it is to unlock your most radiant self.

Prakriti: The Master Blueprint

Prakriti is your unique, inherent constitution, permanently etched into your being at the moment of conception. You might think of it as your body's original code. Modern genetics shows what we carry in our DNA, but Prakriti points to how we actually live and express ourselves in body and mind, the deeper, energetic source code that defines our very nature.

This immutable blueprint remains constant throughout your life, dictating your natural tendencies and defining your original, perfect state of balance. Your **Prakriti** defines your natural, ideal balance of **Doshas** (Vata, Pitta, Kapha) and profoundly influences every facet of your existence, dictating:

- Your Body Type & Metabolism: Your inherent build (slender, medium, sturdy), skin type, hair texture, the efficiency of your digestion (**Agni**), and your natural energy levels.

- Your Mental & Emotional Landscape: Your innate thought patterns, memory capacity, learning style, and typical responses to stress, joy, anger, and fear.
- Your Disease Predispositions: Your unique vulnerabilities and inherent strengths in terms of health and resilience.

By learning to read this blueprint, you gain a powerful lens to proactively manage your health. The profound wisdom that defines this blueprint is captured in a single, powerful shloka from the ancient texts:

"दोषधातुमलमूलं हि शरीरम्"

dosa dhatu mala mūlam hi śariram

(The body is rooted in the Doshas, Dhatus, and Malas.)

This profound statement reveals the three essential components that form the very fabric of your being. They are the core constituents of your **Prakriti** and, when in balance, are the source of your radiant health.

A Forgotten King, A Timeless Message

Understanding your body's blueprint isn't a complex, intellectual exercise; it's about learning to listen to the subtle signals your body gives you. The consequences of not listening are timeless.

Long ago, in a prosperous kingdom, lived a beloved but troubled king. His heart was kind, his rule just, but he was plagued by one unshakable flaw: his unchecked appetite. He did not eat to live; he lived to eat. Meals turned into banquets, snacks into binges. His body grew heavy, his mind dull, and his vitality faded.

One day, the kingdom welcomed Gautam Buddha for a rare sermon. The king, eager to make an impression, ate more than usual to avoid hunger during the discourse. But as Buddha began to speak, the king's overfilled belly lulled him into a deep, shameful slumber.

Seeing this, Buddha quietly walked toward him, gently woke him, and asked, "O King, what has become of you? You, who must protect your people, how will you do so if you cannot protect even your own body?"

The king confessed his addiction, his helplessness before food. Buddha turned to the king's trusted bodyguard,

Chandrashekhar. "You guard the king's body from swords," he said, "but who guards it from his own choices?"

Buddha smiled. "From today, whenever your king eats, gently remind him: 'This is Buddha's message, protect your body, for it is your first kingdom.' Say nothing more. Let that be your only duty."

And so, he did. Day after day, meal after meal, Chandrashekhar's quiet reminder echoed in the king's ears. At first, the king resisted. Then... he paused. Then... he changed. Within days, he grew conscious. Within months, he was transformed. The once-indulgent king stood before Buddha, lighter, sharper, and radiant.

He bowed with folded hands, whispering, "You saved my kingdom by teaching me to govern my first kingdom, my body."

This story is a timeless reminder that true power begins not with conquering lands but with mastering oneself. The king's indulgence was a symptom of a deeper disconnection from his body's blueprint, leading to a profound **Kapha Dosha** imbalance. His salvation came not from a single solution, but from a constant, mindful reminder, a holistic approach to governing his "first kingdom."

The Three Architects: The Doshas

From the nuanced, interconnected dance of the **Pancha Mahabhuta** within you, emerge the three fundamental energetic principles known as **Doshas**. Think of them not as fixed labels, but as the three living forces of your body that guide every physiological and psychological function.

The word 'Dosha' means that which can go wrong when it shifts out of balance. These forces keep the body running, but when disturbed, they become the root of illness.

Vata (Air & Space) – The Principle of Movement. Have you ever felt a headache after a night of poor sleep? Do you sometimes find yourself overthinking, unable to calm your mind? Perhaps you have dry skin in the winter, or your eyes feel strained and parched after too much screen time. Have you noticed joint pains or felt a sudden stomach ache or asthma as the weather turns cloudy and cold?

Why do you think this happens? This is the work of your **Vata Dosha**, the principal force of movement and change in your body. When it goes out of balance, its natural qualities of lightness and mobility turn into restlessness, dryness, and instability.

- **Qualities:** Light, dry, cool, mobile, subtle, quick, rough.

- **Governs:** All movement in the body, from walking and talking to nerve impulses and cellular activity.
- **Imbalance:** Prone to anxiety, restlessness, insomnia, joint pain, constipation, dry skin, and erratic energy.

"वायुतन्त्रधरः प्राणसंग्रहो वायुः शरीराणाम्"

Vayustantra, dharah Prana, samgraho vayuh śariranam
– Charaka Samhita

(Vata is the prime sustainer, the very life force of the body.)

Pitta (Fire & Water) – The Principle of Transformation. Have you ever felt a sharp chest burn after eating a spicy Indian curry? Do you find your eyes become watery or irritated after too much screen time? Have you noticed hyperpigmentation after too much sun exposure, or do you get intensely angry when stressed or irritated? Perhaps you've dealt with cracked heels or irritable bowels every autumn.

Why do you think this happens? This is the work of your **Pitta Dosha**, the powerful force of digestion and transformation. When it goes out of balance, its qualities of heat and intensity manifest as inflammation, irritation, and a feeling of being "burnt out."

- **Qualities:** Hot, sharp, oily, intense, spreading, liquid.
- **Governs:** All transformations: digestion, metabolism, body temperature, hunger, thirst, intellectual capacity, and emotional responses like anger, courage, and discernment.
- **Imbalance:** Prone to irritability, anger, inflammation, acid reflux, skin rashes, and perfectionism.

"पित्तं पाक, ऊष्मा, अग्नि, नीलमञ्जन, शक्ति, वर्णकृत्"

Pittam paka, ūsma, agni, nilamañjana, śakti, varna, krt– *Sushruta Samhita*

(Pitta governs digestion, heat, vision, and complexion.)

Kapha (Water & Earth) – The Principle of Stability. Have you ever felt a heavy, dull feeling after eating a big meal? Do you get sleepy during the day, leading to a heavy-headed feeling? Have you noticed you are more susceptible to coughs and colds every spring, or do you feel numbness in your body if you sit in one place for too long? Do you sometimes lack the motivation to do anything, feeling a deep sense of lethargy?

Why do you think this happens? This is the work of your **Kapha Dosha**, the powerful force of stability and structure.

When it goes out of balance, its qualities of heaviness and slowness lead to stagnation, congestion, and mental dullness.

- **Qualities:** Heavy, slow, cool, moist, smooth, soft, stable, dense, sticky.
- **Governs:** Structure, lubrication, cohesion, and stability: formation of bones and muscles, fluid balance, strength, and immunity.
- **Imbalance:** Prone to lethargy, weight gain, congestion, and attachment.

"कफः शरीरशान्तिबलस्थैर्यात्मकः"

Kaphah Sharira, śanti, bala, sthairya, atmakah–
Ashtanga Hrudayam

(Kapha imparts calmness, strength, and stability to the body.)

While all three **Doshas** are present in everyone, your unique identity arises from the dominance of one, two, or, rarely, all three. Understanding these subtle qualities within your own body is like receiving the personalized manual for your extraordinary design.

The Doshas at Work: Your Tissues and Processes (Dhatus & Malas)

The **Doshas** are the skilled architects and engineers, ceaselessly building and maintaining the very fabric of your body. This form is fundamentally composed of **Dhatus**, the seven essential tissues that support, nourish, and form the structures of your being.

1. **Rasa** (Plasma/Lymph): Liquid nourishment carrying life's essence to every cell.
2. **Rakta** (Blood): The vibrant red fluid carrying oxygen and vitality.
3. **Mamsa** (Muscle): Provides physical strength, movement, and form.
4. **Meda** (Fat): Offers lubrication, insulation, and energy storage.
5. **Asthi** (Bone): Provides the main structure, framework, and unwavering support.
6. **Majja** (Bone Marrow/Nervous Tissue): Fills the bones and is crucial for nerve function.
7. **Shukra** (Reproductive Tissue): The final, most refined tissue, embodying pure vitality and immunity.

These Dhatus are always in motion, each one nourishing the next in a natural sequence, building and maintaining the body's strength. Their health and proper formation are paramount for overall well-being.

Through the continuous processes of digestion and cellular activity, the body naturally creates byproducts. These are the **Malas** (waste products like urine, feces, and sweat). **Malas** are absolutely vital for maintaining balance; they are the body's natural cleansing mechanisms, ensuring that what is no longer needed is efficiently removed. When **Malas** are properly and regularly eliminated, the body remains light, clear, and vibrant. However, when elimination is hindered, these waste products linger, leading to stagnation and discomfort.

Prakriti's Enduring Wisdom: A Personalized Roadmap

Understanding your **Prakriti** offers unparalleled insight into your body because it reveals your inherent strengths and weaknesses, not just a fleeting symptom. This ancient wisdom provides an invaluable roadmap for navigating the complexities of modern living.

Consider an individual with a dominant **Pitta Prakriti**, inherently blessed with strong digestive fire (**Agni**), sharp intellect, and a driven nature. Their natural constitution means their **Pitta Dosha** is naturally high.

If this individual adopts habits that further ignite their inner fire, excessive spicy foods, little rest, or holding onto anger, their **Pitta Dosha** will rapidly accumulate. This heightened **Pitta** can then begin to "cook" or inflame their tissues (**Dhatus**), leading to conditions like skin rashes or acidity.

A skilled **Vaidya** (Ayurvedic practitioner) would recognize these patterns not just as isolated symptoms, but as deeply rooted expressions of their **Prakriti** out of balance. The remedy would be personalized, focusing on cooling and soothing habits, rather than a generic treatment.

This is the profound insight: your **Prakriti** informs your entire physiology and psychology, including your unique predispositions to certain imbalances. By understanding your unique energetic makeup, you gain a powerful lens to proactively manage your health. It's not about finding a cure for a symptom, but about living in harmony with your true self to prevent imbalances from taking root.

For Reflection

1. **Your "First Kingdom":** The story of the king reminds us that true power begins with self-mastery. In what area of your life, your diet, your routines, or your mental habits,

have you been "governed" by a choice that is not serving your highest well-being?

2. **Identifying the "Architect":** Based on the descriptions of **Vata**, **Pitta**, and **Kapha**, which **Dosha** seems most dominant in your core nature when you are at your best? And which one is most out of balance when you are feeling unwell?
3. **The Silent Signals:** What is one subtle sign of imbalance (**Vikriti**) that your body has been sending you lately (e.g., a feeling of restlessness, irritability, or lethargy)? How can you use the three **Dosha** descriptions to better understand what this signal is telling you?
4. **A Personalized Rhythm:** The chapter speaks of your **Prakriti** as a blueprint. What is one habit or lifestyle choice you can make this week that is in direct alignment with your natural constitution, as opposed to a generic health trend?

Action Plan: Your Daily Blueprint

This is not a one-day detox. Ayurveda insists on consistency. Your daily rhythm is your medicine. The **Doshas**, **Dhatus**, and **Malas** stay aligned only when you:

- Sleep, wake, and eat with regularity.

- Support digestion daily (**Agni** is king).
- Practice moderation, not extremes.

These aren't just short-term tips. They are simple, steady practices that can become anchors for your health over a lifetime.

Cheat Sheet 1: Aligning with Your Dosha (Your Lifetime Rhythm Anchors)

Vata Dosha (Air + Space)

- **3 Things to DO**
  1. **Maintain a Grounding Routine (Dinacharya: An ayurvedic routine):** Wake, eat, and sleep at consistent times each day to create stability.
  2. **Favor Warm, Nourishing Foods:** Prioritize warm, cooked meals with healthy fats like **ghee** and sesame oil. Spices like ginger, cinnamon, and cardamom are essential.
  3. **Practice Soothing Rituals:** Engage in **Abhyanga** (daily self-oil massage) with warm sesame oil and calm, intentional breathing like **Nadi Shodhana** (Alternate Nostril Breathing).

- **3 Things to AVOID**
    1. **Irregularity and Rushing:** Avoid skipping meals, erratic sleep schedules, and excessive travel.
    2. **Cold, Dry, and Raw Foods:** Reduce intake of salads, crackers, cold drinks, and ice cream.
    3. **Overstimulation:** Limit screen time, loud environments, and late-night activities.

Pitta Dosha (Fire + Water)

- **3 Things to DO**
    1. **Embrace the Cooling and Calming:** Incorporate cooling foods like cucumber, mint, cilantro, and coconut. Use sweet, astringent, and bitter tastes in your diet.
    2. **Cultivate a Cool Head:** Practice cooling **Pranayama** like **Sheetali** (Sipping Breath) and **Brahmari** (Humming Bee Breath). Spend time near cool water or in the moonlight.
    3. **Release Control:** Engage in non-competitive, calming activities. Learn to delegate and avoid heated arguments and perfectionism.

- **3 Things to AVOID**
    1. **Heat-Inducing Foods:** Stay away from excessive spicy, sour, and fried foods.
    2. **Overwork and Conflict:** Avoid skipping meals, holding onto anger, and pushing yourself to the point of burnout.
    3. **Excessive Sun and Heat:** Limit direct sun exposure during midday and avoid alcohol.

Kapha Dosha (Water + Earth)

- **3 Things to DO**
    1. **Awaken to Movement:** Rise early, preferably before sunrise (**Brahma Muhurta**). Begin your day with brisk movement like walking, hiking, or an energetic yoga sequence.
    2. **Favor Light, Pungent Foods:** Include foods that are light, warm, and spicy to stimulate digestion (**Agni**). Use spices like ginger, black pepper, and chili.
    3. **Cultivate a Disciplined Mind:** Engage in new activities regularly to avoid stagnation. Practice invigorating breathing like **Bhastrika** (Bellows Breath) to clear congestion.

- **3 Things to AVOID**
    1. **Heavy, Oily, and Sweet Foods:** Limit intake of dairy, fried foods, and excessive sugar.
    2. **Sluggish Habits:** Avoid daytime naps, especially after meals, and prolonged periods of inactivity.
    3. **Emotional Stagnation:** Release emotional attachments and avoid holding onto possessions.

Closing Note: Embracing Your Divine Design

Your Prakriti is your unique blend of energies, shaping how you are at your core. It isn't a limit; it's a guide to how you can live in your best rhythm. By understanding and honoring this blueprint, you step into a powerful partnership with your own body, aligning with the deepest truths of your being.

This is a step toward self-understanding. When you know your Prakriti, you can make choices, in food, in routine, even in thought, that support your well-being more naturally. In the chapters to come, we will explore the practical tools and daily rhythms, informed by your unique **Prakriti**, that will allow you to consciously bring your **Sharira** into its most harmonious state, protecting you from imbalance and unleashing your true potential.

“शरीरमाद्यंखलु धर्मसाधनम्”

Shariramadyam khalu dharmasadhanam

(The body is the first tool to fulfill your soul’s purpose.)

Summary

- **Discover your unique Prakriti:** Uncover the innate, energetic blueprint that shapes your body, mind, and lifelong tendencies.
- **Meet the Doshas:** Learn how **Vata**, **Pitta**, and **Kapha** orchestrate your constitution, physical health, and personality, each influencing you in subtle, powerful ways.
- **Understand Dhatus and Malas:** Grasp the crucial roles of your body’s tissues and elimination processes in sustaining wellness and vitality.
- **Spot imbalances:** Recognize the telltale signs when **Doshas** drift from balance, and how they impact your energy, mood, and resilience.
- **Turn insight into practice:** Reflect on your own tendencies, and choose food, lifestyle, and self-care rituals that truly fit your personal nature.

- **Begin with breath:** Use accessible tools like **Pranayama** to rebalance and harmonize your **Doshas** every day.
- **Step toward self-care**: Honoring your original design creates the ground for health, steadiness, and the joy of living true to yourself.

Chapter 5:

The Life Energy Within: Prana, Agni, and the Spark of Life

"प्राणिनां प्रथमं प्राणः।"

Praninam prathamam Pranah. – Ayurveda Sutra

*(Among all the vital forces, **Prana** is primary.)*

In the previous chapter, we unveiled **Prakriti** (unique, original constitution), your unique blueprint for how the **Pancha Mahabhuta** (five great elements) manifest into the **Doshas** (**Vata**, **Pitta**, **Kapha**), orchestrating the formation of **Dhatus** (tissues) and the elimination of **Malas** (wastes). We saw that your **Prakriti** is your fixed, ideal state, while **Vikriti** (a state of imbalance) reflects your dynamic imbalances, offering a personalized roadmap to health. Now, we dive deeper into the very forces that animate this intricate design, giving it life, consciousness, and the power to thrive.

You are not only flesh and bone. You are breath, energy, and the quiet rhythms that keep you alive moment to moment. If the body is an instrument, Prana is the breath that moves it, Agni the fire that powers it, and Ojas the quiet strength it preserves. To know them is not just to understand health, it is to awaken to the miracle of being alive.

Have you ever watched a social media video of an Indian soldier, stationed high in the Himalayan snows, who sees a man walking barefoot, clad only in a simple cloth? The astonished soldier asks the man, "Are you not feeling cold?" The man replies with a simple serenity, "Shiva is taking care of me." What allows a human to transcend the ordinary limits of the physical body? The answer lies in the subtle energy within.

This is the very essence of **Prana** (life force), the vital energy that animates your body. While we have limited resources, a few people possess the capacity to truly harness this powerful force. This is the same vital energy referred to as **Chi** in Chinese medicine or **Zen** in Buddhist traditions. Your body, made of **Pancha Mahabhuta**, **Prakriti**, **Dosha**, **Dhatus**, and **Malas** as seen in previous chapters, would be lifeless without the animating power of **Prana** and **Agni** (digestive fire).

You might think of **Prana** as just oxygen and **Agni** as just metabolism, but they are far more profound. **Prana** is the very intelligence that governs the breath, while **Agni** is the power to produce and harness this energy. Ultimately, to understand their importance, simply consider this: remove them, and there is no life. Any blockage in the flow of **Prana** will lead to profound effects. Think of your erratic breathing during stress, and you will understand why controlling **Prana** is so crucial. That process of conscious control is **Pranayama** (breath control), the core concept of mindful living, which grants you command over both your body and your mental state. A weak **Agni**, on the other hand, can lead to numerous problems and block the subtle energy channels of the body. Together, they are the very foundation of your vitality.

The Body's Orchestra: Prana, Agni, and Ojas

Imagine your body not as a machine, but as a living community. Trillions of cells each play their role, and together they create harmony. This silent coordination, this shared rhythm, is the signature of life itself. When this harmony breaks, we call it a disease of disunity, a profound dissonance orchestrated when life's subtle energies become deeply distorted.

What fuels this symphony? These trillions of cells draw their energy from the great inner furnace, **Agni**. And to coordinate this entire community, we need communication, a sacred electricity that informs, connects, and unites. This spark is **Prana**.

"**Agni** gives you the fuel. **Prana** gives you the signal."

Together, Agni and Prana keep life steady. But when we weaken Agni with careless eating and disturb Prana with restless minds, even rest can leave us tired.

We chase energy in caffeine and sugar, while the true sources, breath, balance, and inner fire, lie waiting, neglected.

Prana: The Cosmic Current

“प्राणेन रक्षते सर्वम् जगत् सर्वं यत् किञ्चित् प्राणे प्रतिष्ठितम्।”

Pranena raksate sarvam jagat sarvam yat kiñcit prane pratisthitam. – Brhadaranyaka Upanisad

(All that exists in the universe is sustained by Prana, for all that moves is established in Prana.)

Prana is the universal life force that animates everything. It’s more than just oxygen; it is the breath within the breath, the intelligence that moves life itself, flowing through your **Nadis** (subtle energy channels). Think of Nadis as invisible rivers of energy, like Wi-Fi signals carrying life through your body, the subtle energy channels that weave your inner cosmos. There are 72000 Nadis in the human body. When these channels are open, **Prana** flows freely, bringing health, clarity, and vitality.

Prana in Real Life: Meet Alex, a young mountaineer who froze in panic on a sheer rock face. Through his breathwork, he regained control, calming his mind and body. This conscious control of his breath allowed **Prana** to flow, guiding him safely to the summit and revealing a new level of inner strength.

Reflect: When was the last time you felt your own **Prana** pulse with possibility? Or a day when your breath was shallow and you felt disconnected from your own body?

The Great Conversation: An Ancient Tale

Once, the five senses, sight, sound, taste, touch, and smell, along with the mind, gathered for a great debate. They argued over which among them was the most essential to the body's existence.

The eye declared, "Without me, the world is a dark void! I am the most vital." The ear protested, "No! Without me, there is only deafening silence. I am supreme!" The tongue boasted, "I am the source of all pleasure and sustenance!" The mind, swelling with pride, proclaimed, "I am the rulcr of all! Without me, senses are meaningless!"

They bickered for days, each convinced of its own supremacy. Finally, **Prana**, who had remained silent until then, decided to leave the body. As **Prana** began to depart, the senses started to lose their power. The eye's vision dimmed, the ear's hearing faded, and the mind's thoughts scattered. Life itself began to ebb away. In a moment of sheer panic, the senses and the mind cried out for **Prana** to return.

"Oh, glorious **Prana**! You are indeed the most essential," they pleaded. "Without you, we are but empty vessels. We are all sustained by you."

And so, **Prana** returned, restoring life, clarity, and vitality to the senses and the mind.

This ancient story, from the **Upanisads** (ancient Sanskrit texts of spiritual teaching and ideas), teaches a profound truth: all of our functions—our senses, our thoughts, our actions—are dependent on the flow of **Prana**. It is the life-giving energy that underlies every biological process. It is the breath of God within us.

Modern Analogy: The Battery of Your Being

In our modern world, we understand the concept of energy through technology. Consider **Prana** as your body's battery. Every action, a thought, a feeling, a physical movement, affects your Prana. When your **Prana** is high, you feel vibrant, focused, and resilient. When it's low, you feel fatigued, stressed, and easily overwhelmed.

Our modern lifestyle is a drain on this battery. Chronic stress, poor sleep, processed foods, and a lack of connection to nature deplete our **Prana** rapidly. We've become a society running on empty, trying to function with a battery at 10%.

The path of **Sukh-Arogyam** (the harmonious union of easeful joy and radiant wellness) teaches us how to recharge this battery. By consciously cultivating **Prana** through simple practices, we can restore our vitality, build our resilience, and awaken the deep inner strength that is our birthright.

Agni: The Sacred Fire Within

"अग्निर्मूर्धा दिवः ककुत्पतिः पृथिव्या अयम्।"

Agnir mūrdha divah kakut patih prthivya ayam. – Atharva Veda

(Agni is the head of the heavens, the pinnacle of the earth.)

The Sanskrit word **Agni** (अग्नि), for "fire," is your inner alchemist, the hearth fire that transforms raw food into nourishment, fleeting thoughts into wisdom, and life's chaos into clarity. Its heart is **Jatharagni** (digestive fire), the digestive flame in your gut. Subtler fires, **Bhutagnis** (elemental fires) for the elements and **Dhatu Agnis** (tissue fires) for your tissues, carry their spark to every cell.

Agni is not just the fire in your stomach; it is present in every tissue, every cell, and every psychological process. It is the wisdom that converts food into nourishment, sensory information into knowledge, and emotions into experience.

Think of **Agni** as the gatekeeper of health. It is the force that separates what is useful from what is waste. A strong **Agni** ensures that your body absorbs nutrients, destroys pathogens, and eliminates toxins effectively. A weak **Agni** leads to the accumulation of **Ama** (आम), a sticky, toxic residue that clogs the channels of the body and is the root cause of most diseases.

Agni in Everyday Life: A corporate executive, Mark, was plagued by bloat and mental fog after lunch. He discovered mindful eating and simple **Agni**-building rituals. By eating his largest meal at noon and pausing to bless his food, his digestion improved, and his mind became sharp and clear again.

Reflect: Think of a meal you ate today. Did you eat mindfully and feel nourished? Or did you eat quickly and feel drained afterward?

A Story of Two Brothers

In a small village, there lived two brothers, Varun and Rohan. Varun was cautious and ate simple, easily digestible meals at the same time every day. He favored warm, spiced foods and never overate. Rohan, on the other hand, was an adventurer. He would eat anything at any time, spicy street food, heavy sweets late at night, and cold drinks with every meal.

Varun had a clear mind, a strong body, and rarely fell ill. He possessed a serene inner glow that made him beloved by all. Rohan, despite his adventurous spirit, was often plagued by indigestion, lethargy, and a constant feeling of mental fog. His skin was dull, and his energy was erratic.

One day, a wise **Vaidya** (Ayurvedic physician) visited the village. Both brothers went to him for guidance. The **Vaidya** looked at Varun and said, "Your **Agni** is bright. You honor the inner fire, and in return, it sustains your body and mind." He then turned to Rohan and said, "Your inner fire is dim and choked with undigested food. You have created **Ama** (toxins), and it has dampened your vitality."

The **Vaidya** explained that the same food that nourished Varun was creating toxins in Rohan because of his weakened **Agni**. He advised Rohan to treat his digestion like a sacred fire, to feed it with care, to avoid dousing it with cold water, and to never overburden it.

Rohan, humbled by the lesson, began to follow the **Vaidya's** advice. Slowly, his vitality returned, and his mind became clear. He realized that the greatest adventure was not in conquering the world, but in mastering the fire within.

This story illustrates a core Ayurvedic truth: In truth, it's not only what we eat that matters, but what the body can actually digest and use. The state of our **Agni** determines our ability to transform, nourish, and eliminate.

Ojas, Tejas, and Sattva – The Subtle Triad of Vitality

This trio represents the refined essences of your immunity, clarity, and peace of mind. They are the golden glow of true health.

Ojas: The Inner Reservoir of Immunity and Joy **Ojas** is the final product of perfect digestion, the essence of immunity, emotional steadiness, and profound vitality.

- **Signs of Strength:**
  - Luminous vitality and a natural glow
  - Sustained energy and strong immunity
  - A calm, stable, and resilient disposition
- **Signs of Depletion:**
  - Frequent illness and chronic fatigue
  - Emotional instability and burnout
  - Dull skin and eyes **Ojas**'

Secret: Grandma Lila never gets sick, and at 85, she radiates joy. Her secret isn't complicated: she gets a full night's sleep, eats simple, nourishing food, and ends each day with gratitude, cultivating her **Ojas** and keeping her inner light shining bright. **Reflect:** When you feel your best, what does that feel like? And when was the last time you felt your immunity was truly strong?

Tejas: The Radiance of Being **Tejas** is the luster of your inner fire, the subtle energetic spark of **Agni** in the mind and body. It governs metabolic clarity, cellular energy, and spiritual vitality.

- **Signs of Strength:**

    - Radiant presence and keen intellect
    - Courage and decisive action
    - Sharp, focused awareness
- **Signs of Depletion:**
    - Brain fog and dull skin
    - Indecision and a lack of willpower
    - Fatigue and a feeling of "burnout" **Tejas** and

Creativity: When artist Meera lost her creative drive, her colors faded, and her mind felt cloudy. A simple daily walk in the sunlight and a moment of stillness each morning rekindled her **Tejas**. Her energy, ideas, and confidence returned as if a veil had been lifted. **Reflect:** When did you last feel a surge of creative energy or a moment of profound mental clarity?

Sattva: The Mind's Inner Light **Sattva** is the purest quality of the mind, reflecting clarity, emotional intelligence, and spiritual stability.

- **Signs of Strength:**
    - Inner peace and profound resilience
    - Natural compassion and clear judgment
    - A calm, balanced state of mind
- **Signs of Depletion:**
    - Mental agitation and confusion

- Aggression, depression, or lethargy
- Being easily swayed by intense emotions **Sattva** in a Parent:

Ryen, a busy parent, discovered that his daily 10-minute meditation practice brought him more than just personal calm. It gave him the patience and kindness to navigate his children's tantrums with compassion, permeating the lives of his whole family. **Reflect:** How often do you feel a sense of inner peace, even when chaos surrounds you?

When Harmony is Disturbed

When **Prana** is blocked, **Agni** is dim, and **Ojas** is depleted, everything in life feels the strain. We rush through meals, eat late, sleep irregularly, overstimulate our minds with screens, and ignore our emotional digestion. These habits not only disturb **Agni** but also block the **Nadis**, dulling the flow of **Prana**. This disconnect creates cracks in our vitality.

Over time, this neglect erodes **Ojas**, the essence of immunity and resilience. You feel more fatigued, more reactive, less protected. The glow fades. When **Ojas** diminishes, so does **Tejas**, your inner radiance. The eyes lose their spark. The mind becomes foggy. The spirit feels dim. And when **Tejas** dims, **Sattva** struggles. Your inner peace is drowned in noise, your judgment clouded, your spirit restless.

You might not be a wandering sage or an artist seeking sunlight, but the vital spark of **Prana**, **Agni**, and **Ojas** is your birthright, too. How will you choose to nurture it today?

For Reflection

1. **The Agni-Ama Connection:** The chapter shares the story of Varun and Rohan, highlighting how a weak **Agni** can create **Ama**. Think about your own daily habits. What is one "cold drink" (an activity, a food, or a thought) that you regularly use that might be dampening your inner fire? What is one small, warm, mindful choice you can make to kindle it?
2. **Prana and Your Inner Dialogue:** The story of the senses reminds us that **Prana** is the foundation of all function, including the mind. When your mind is at its most chaotic, perhaps during stress or anxiety, how does your breathing change? How can the conscious act of taking a deep, calming breath interrupt that chaos and reconnect you to your inner **Prana**?
3. **The Fading Glow:** The chapter explains that neglecting **Agni** and **Prana** can erode **Ojas**, dimming **Tejas** and weakening **Sattva**. Look at the signs of strength and

depletion for each of these. Which of these three subtle essences do you feel is most in need of your attention right now? What is one simple ritual you can adopt to nourish it?

4. **Beyond the Obvious:** We often think of **Agni** only in terms of food. But it also digests our experiences and emotions. Consider a challenging event you went through recently. Did you "digest" it fully, or are you still holding onto it? What is one way you can release this undigested emotional residue to free up your inner fire?

Actionable Plan: Rekindling Your Inner Light

The path of **Sukh-Arogyam** (the harmonious union of easeful joy and radiant wellness) is one of profound reverence for the body's wisdom. By honoring the fire within, you not only improve your digestion but also empower your mind, strengthen your immunity, and illuminate your spiritual purpose. Your **Agni** is the sacred flame that sustains your entire being. Nurture it, and you will live a life of radiant health and vibrant energy.

This is not a quick fix. It's a steady practice, and its benefits deepen over time.

Action 1: Pranayama as a Tool for Balance

The breath is the most direct bridge between your mind and body, a powerful tool for self-regulation and balancing the **Doshas**. Conscious breathing practices, known as **Pranayama**, can calm a restless **Vata** mind, cool an overheated **Pitta** system, or energize a sluggish **Kapha** body. Begin with these two simple techniques to start your journey of inner harmony.

Nadi Shodhana Pranayama (Alternate Nostril Breathing)

This is a foundational practice for calming the nervous system and balancing the three **Doshas**. It cleanses and harmonizes the subtle energy channels (**Nadis**) of the body, bringing clarity and peace.

- **How to Practice:**
    1. Sit comfortably with a straight spine.
    2. Gently close your right nostril with your right thumb.
    3. Inhale slowly and deeply through your left nostril.
    4. Close the left nostril with your ring finger, release the thumb, and exhale through the right nostril.
    5. Inhale through the right nostril.

6. Close the right nostril, release the ring finger, and exhale through the left nostril.
7. This completes one round. Continue for 5-10 rounds.

Brahmari Pranayama (Humming Bee Breath) This practice is especially effective for soothing a busy mind and cooling an overheated system. The gentle humming sound creates an internal vibration that calms the nervous system and promotes deep relaxation.

- **How to Practice:**
    1. Sit comfortably with a straight spine.
    2. Close your ears with your thumbs and place your index fingers over your eyes.
    3. Take a deep, slow inhale through your nose.
    4. As you exhale, keep your mouth closed and make a soft, humming sound like a bee.
    5. Continue for 5-7 breaths. Notice the calming vibration throughout your head and chest.

Action 2: Authentic Agni Rituals

These aren't quick tricks, but time-honored practices that stoke your inner fire.

1. **Sip Warm Water:** Start your day with a glass of warm water. This simple act gently cleanses the digestive

tract and awakens your **Agni** without shocking it. It's the most authentic way to honor your digestive fire.

2. **Use Agni-Kindling Spices:** Before your main meal, try a small piece of fresh ginger with a pinch of rock salt and a few drops of fresh lime juice. This simple "appetizer" awakens the digestive enzymes and prepares your stomach to receive food.
3. **Honor the Sun's Rhythm:** Eat your largest meal when your digestive fire is naturally at its peak: midday. Have a lighter, earlier dinner. This aligns your internal fire with the sun's rhythm, which is the cosmic reflection of **Agn**

Remember, these simple practices, breathing with awareness, honouring your Agni with warmth, eating in rhythm with the sun, are not the whole journey. They light the way into a larger journey called **Sukh-Arogyam**.

Bridge to Chapter 6: The Roots of Imbalance

These five currents, **Prana**, **Agni**, **Ojas**, **Tejas**, and **Sattva**, form the essence of your **Sharira**'s (physical body) health, vitality, and consciousness. They are meant to flow in perfect harmony, but your fire may flicker, your breath may falter, your clarity may dim. These are not random occurrences;

they are signals. They stem from your daily rituals, your environment, your conscious (or unconscious) choices, and even profound cosmic influences.

Next chapter is how your body gets into problem and roots of problem.

Chapter 6:

The Roots of Disease – Dosha Imbalance and Ama

"रोगास्तु दोषविषमसमन्विता

rogastu dosa-visama-samanvitah– Charaka Samhita

Disease is born from the conjunction of imbalanced Doshas.

In the last chapter, we awakened to the miracle of **Prana** (life force) and **Agni** (digestive fire), the luminous dance of breath and fire that powers your **Sharira** (physical body). We learned how these vital forces give you life, energy, and clarity. Yet, even these brilliant energies dim when we ignore their subtle calls to balance. This brings us to the silent, gradual birth of disease, a process that doesn't happen in a moment, but over many days of ignored whispers.

Sudden Collapse—Silent Warnings of a Tired World

Just days ago, headlines broke of a young woman, radiant, laughing, lost in the joy of dance at a wedding, who collapsed mid-performance and never woke again. A schoolgirl, moments before playing with her friends, suddenly fell to the ground and was no more. These aren't isolated events. Every week, every feed, every scroll whispers of lives cut short.

We look at these tragedies and say: “So sudden.” But were they, really?

Disease never arrives in a single day; it gives subtle signs. It grows, quietly, relentlessly, through tiny breaches of balance, one unnoticed signal at a time. The ache was ignored. The sleep was skipped. The emotions were buried. The smile worn like armor while something inside silently corrodes. We cover pain with pills. We override fatigue with caffeine. We normalize burnout. But the body always speaks before it screams. Are you listening?

Disease Does Not Just Happen — It Grows from Disrespect

Disease does not knock loudly at first. It whispers in skipped meals, repressed emotions, and sleepless nights. It is born not of chance, but of subtle disregard, a forgetfulness of your body’s sacred rhythm, of the balance that sustains you. Disease is less an enemy than a result of forgetting, forgetting rhythm, balance, and care for the different parts of our life.

At the root of almost every disorder, physical, emotional, and mental, are two ancient saboteurs: **Dosha** imbalance and **Ama**. While **Doshas** are the elemental forces that govern your being, **Ama** is the sticky residue, physical, emotional, mental, that accumulates when these forces are misused. One disturbs, the other clogs. Together, they create the perfect storm for disease.

When Your Inner Architects Go Rogue – The Dosha Drama

Your **Doshas**, **Vata**, **Pitta**, and **Kapha**, are the fundamental intelligences of the body. These Doshas guide all functions of the body. When in balance, they support harmony; when disturbed, they bring discomfort and disease. But if a string is too tight, it snaps with tension and irritability. If too loose, it sags, losing its vibrant melody. Similarly, your **Doshas** are dynamic, and they do not tolerate neglect.

When you disrespect your **Sharira** (body), **Manas** (mind), **Bhava** (emotion), **Sambandh** (relationships), **Dhan** (wealth/work), or **Paryavaran** (environment), your **Doshas** become agitated. They no longer build, they sabotage.

Let's look at how each **Dosha** rebels:

Vata in Uproar (Air & Space Gone Wild)

- **Disrespectful Triggers:** Late nights (**Sharira**), chronic worry (**Manas**), Multitasking without rest (**Manas**), Skipping meals (**Sharira**), isolation (**Sambandh**), Digital overload (**Paryavaran**)
- **Manifestations:** Anxiety, insomnia, constipation, joint pain, nerve sensitivity/disorders, chronic fatigue.

It feels like a windy storm inside, a hurricane without having any grounding.

Pitta on Fire (Blaze Out of Control)

- **Disrespectful Triggers:** Overuse of spicy, junk fried foods (**Sharira**), suppressed anger or constant criticism (**Bhava**), Relentless work pace (**Dhan/Manas**), High, heat environments (**Paryavaran**).
- **Manifestations:** Acid reflux, ulcers, inflammatory skin conditions, liver problems, early greying, intense anger.

Like a fire spreading too quickly, Pitta out of balance consumes the calm of body and mind.

Kapha in Stagnation (Earth & Water Overwhelmed)

- **Disrespectful Triggers:** Overeating heavy, sweet, cold foods (**Sharira**), long-held sadness or emotional clinging (**Bhava**), Sedentary lifestyle, purposelessness (**Aatma**), Damp, cluttered spaces (**Paryavaran**)
- **Manifestations:** Weight gain, sinus congestion, diabetes, depression, lethargy, asthma.

A stagnant pond that is dense, dull, and fully overgrown. Needing serious cleaning.

Self-Inquiry Prompt: Think of a recurring health issue you face. Can you identify the **Dosha** at play? What daily act of neglect may be feeding it?

Ama – The Sludge that Silences Vitality

"मन्दोअग्निःसर्वकारणं रोगे। ततःसम्पद्यतेअग्निमान्द्यम्।"

Mando-agnih sarva-karanam roge. Tatah-sampadyate agni-mandyam. – Charaka Samhita

(*A weak fire is the cause of all disease. From this arises the lack of fire.*)

When **Doshas** rebel, they dim **Agni**, birthing **Ama**, the silent sludge that chokes your vitality. **Ama** is the sticky, toxic residue that clings to the body's inner pathways.

The Silent Cost of Greatness – A Tale of Siddharth and the River's Revelation

In ancient India, Prince Siddharth left behind his palace of silk and song to search for truth. He walked through forests, sat beneath trees, and practiced extreme penance. He ate almost nothing. He slept on bare ground. He punished his Sharira, believing that only by weakening the body could the soul be freed.

Years passed, and so did his strength. His Agni, the sacred digestive fire, dimmed to embers. What food he took no longer nourished but lingered half-digested, turning to Ama, the sticky residue of undigested life. His frame grew frail, his eyes lost their luster, and his mind, instead of becoming clear, swirled with fog.

One day, while crossing a river, his weakened body collapsed. The current dragged him under. Breath faltered. Agni had nearly gone out. A stranger pulled him to safety, and there, on the bank, a village girl offered a simple bowl of kheer. At first, Siddharth resisted, his mind still bound by the idea that denying the body was noble. But as he looked at her, he felt another truth stirring:

He realized: "How can truth be seen through eyes blurred by hunger? How can wisdom shine when Agni is extinguished?"

With trembling hands, he accepted. The sweetness of that food rekindled his fire. His body warmed, his mind cleared, and his spirit lifted. Soon after, he sat beneath the Bodhi tree and awakened, not by destroying the body, but by honoring its balance. He became the Buddha, whole, alive, radiant.

The lesson is timeless: fasting beyond need, neglecting nourishment, or punishing the body does not purify, it weakens Agni, breeds Ama, and clouds the light of truth. Balance sustains. Balance liberates.

Then Compact Teaching (transitioning back into Ama theme):

When Agni is dimmed, whether by excess, neglect, or extremes, Ama takes hold. It clogs the body's channels, dulls vitality, and begins to spread silently. This is why Ayurveda warns: disease is not born in a day. It is born in the daily choices that either honor Agni or insult it.

The Clogged Drain

Imagine your body as a magnificent, flowing river. The water is clear, vibrant, and moves effortlessly, carrying nourishment to every cell. This is the state of balance and health. Now, imagine someone begins throwing trash into the river, unhealthy food, stressful emotions, too much stimulation, and too little rest.

At first, the river's current is strong, and it manages to push the debris through. But over time, the trash accumulates. It gets stuck on rocks and banks, forming a stagnant, putrid sludge. That build-up, that heaviness in the river, is what Ayurveda calls Ama.

As Buddha wisely noted, "Clarity comes when the mind is cleansed of what it doesn't need." **Ama** is exactly what the mind and body don't need.

Ama vs. Agni: A Lifelong Tug-of-War

Ama and **Agni** are in a constant, delicate balance. They are like a seesaw. When **Agni** is strong, it burns up any potential **Ama** and maintains your health. When **Agni** is weak, even a small amount of improper food or emotion can lead to the creation of **Ama**. The goal of an Ayurvedic lifestyle is not just to avoid **Ama**, but to build an **Agni** so strong that **Ama** cannot take hold.

The Slug Inside – A Story of Ama

One day, you were just doing your job. You felt a little hungry, but the task at hand was more urgent. "I'll eat in a bit," you told yourself. An hour passed. Your stomach had quieted, and the sharp call of hunger softened into background noise.

Later, you remembered, "Oh, I haven't eaten." So you did. Heavily. Because after all, you'd skipped lunch. Your body wasn't prepared. Your digestive fire, **Agni**, had dimmed in the wait. **The heavy meal sat like a stone, your gut churning, your mind clouded by a fog that stole your spark.**

Your body tried. It always does. But it couldn't break everything down. Some nutrients went unused. Some food remained half-digested. This partially processed mass, sticky, heavy, and unrefined, didn't just disappear. It stayed. It lingered. And slowly, silently, it began to spread.

And so this half-burnt matter, the **Ama**, kept building. Day after day. Skipped hunger cues. Improper meals. Suppressed emotions. No movement. No sweat. No elimination. Your body, the brilliant self-cleaning system it is, tried to sweep the floors. It always does. But even the best cleaners can only do so much if the mess keeps piling.

You didn't notice the early signs. A little heaviness. A little brain fog. A little fatigue. But who has time to notice, right?

You have a life to live. Deadlines to meet. Messages to answer. Content to consume.

So you carried on.

And so did the **Ama**.

This residue, this undigested physical and emotional matter, kept traveling. It began to clog the channels. It looked for weak spots: A sluggish liver. A stressed nervous system. A weakened gut. A tired uterus. A burnt-out brain. And when it found them, it settled. And there, it bloomed into symptoms.

Conditions like PCOS, IBS, diabetes, or anxiety are not random; they often reflect deeper imbalance and a fire that has been dimmed.

This is **Ama**. The toxic residue of undigested life. Not just food, but emotions, thoughts, experiences, and traumas. Everything we couldn't fully process clings. And all of it has one common root: weakened **Agni**. The dimmed digestive fire. The scattered inner flame. The forgotten intelligence of the body.

Pause: Where do you notice this slow build-up in your own body or mind? What's one early warning you normally ignore?

Ama's Manifestations Across the 7 Petals of Sukh-Arogyam

Petal	Expression of **Ama**
Sharira	Fatigue, constipation, dull skin, aches, body odor
Manas	Brain fog, indecision, mental dullness
Bhava	Suppressed emotions, resentment, emotional heaviness
Sambandh	Toxic relationships, superficial bonds, withdrawal
Dhan	Burnout, poor decisions, overworking, stagnation
Paryavaran	Feeling overwhelmed by pollution, clutter, and disconnection
Aatma	Lack of purpose, spiritual disconnection, lethargy

आम मूलं रोगाणाम् "

Ama mūlam roganam"

Ama is the root of all disease.

Beyond these broad manifestations, **Ama** specifically targets and disrupts the proper functioning of various organ systems, causing symptoms that Western medicine often treats in isolation:

- **Digestive System:** Persistent coating on the tongue, foul breath, sluggish bowels, irregular appetite.
- **Circulatory System:** Sticky, impure blood, reduced nutrient delivery, poor circulation, cold extremities.
- **Musculoskeletal System:** Stiffness, joint pain (especially in the morning), body heaviness.
- **Respiratory System:** Chronic cough, sticky phlegm, chest congestion.
- **Nervous & Mental Systems:** Poor memory, mental dullness, brain fog, fatigue unrelieved by rest.
- **Skin:** Dull, oily, or reactive skin prone to rashes or breakouts.

Signs You Can See and Feel: The Whisper of Ama

Ama isn't always hidden. Your body often whispers its presence:

- Thick, white/yellow coat on tongue (especially in the mornings)
- Persistent body odor
- Heavy, dull, sticky sensation, especially upon waking

- Dull skin, clammy, or oily
- Joint stiffness/aches, irritable in damp/cold
- Digestive irregularity, incomplete elimination

Through **Nadi Pariksha** (pulse diagnosis), tongue/eye/nail reading, and conversation, an Ayurvedic expert sees these "whispers" as clear maps of disorder and imbalance.

The Storm, the Sludge, and the Garden

Imagine **Dosha** imbalance as a storm, **Vata**'s erratic winds dry your skin and create internal turbulence, **Pitta**'s intense heat scorches your gut and fuels inflammation, and **Kapha**'s heavy rain floods your energy and leads to stagnation. Into this storm, **Ama** enters as the sludge, more than just physical toxins, it's undigested life (be it food, emotions, or thoughts) that clogs your vibrant inner river, dulling the very shine of your **Dhatus** (tissues).

Ayurveda teaches that we must clear this **Ama** first, like weeding a garden before watering. Only then can your **Sharira** truly bloom, vibrant and alive. This profound connection between your subtle energies, accumulated **Ama**, and overall well-being is strongly supported by both Ayurveda's **Tridosha** principles and modern understanding of immunology and systemic inflammation.

The Cycle of Disrespect → Dosha Imbalance → Ama → Disease

One small act of disrespect to a single petal can begin a domino effect:

- Eat heavy food late → **Kapha** rises
- Weak **Agni** → **Ama** forms
- You wake up heavy and foggy → You skip morning yoga
- Stagnant **Prana** → Fatigued **Manas**
- Clouded thoughts → Poor decisions

It's not about blame. It is simply cause and effect, and the reminder that we have the choice to act differently.

Case Study: Sunita, the Overachiever But this isn't just theory. Let's meet Sunita, a real-life reflection of modern imbalance. Sunita, 42, ran a startup with passion but no pause. She skipped meals, slept late, worked weekends. Her **Doshas** rebelled. Her **Agni** collapsed. **Ama** built up, manifesting as chronic fatigue, bloating, and mood swings. When she returned to rest, mindful meals, and daily movement, her digestion improved, her glow returned, and her joy in work re-emerged.

The Modern Parallel: Inflammation – Ama in Scientific Language

Even Western medicine now echoes this ancient insight. Chronic inflammation is their word for what Ayurveda calls **Ama**.

> *"Inflammation is the root of most chronic disease." – Dr. Andrew Weil*

Inflammation = **Ama** + **Agni** Disturbance. It's the smoldering fire that never fully burns, quietly corroding vitality.

For Reflection

1. **The Fading Glow:** We often ignore the first whispers of **Ama**. Where do you notice a dullness or lack of clarity in your own life—in your skin, your mind, or your energy? What's one consistent habit (physical or mental) that you suspect is causing this?
2. **The Undigested Emotion:** The chapter mentions that **Ama** can be emotional. Think of a long-held grudge or a stressful experience that you haven't fully processed. How does that "stuck" emotion physically manifest for you? (e.g., in your gut, your shoulders, or a headache).
3. **The Three Doors of Ama: Ama** enters through your senses, your food, and your thoughts. Consider your day yesterday. What did you consume (food, news, social

media, etc.) that may have weakened your **Agni** and contributed to the accumulation of **Ama**?

4. **Aatma's Connection:** How has **Ama** dulled your spiritual connection (**Aatma**)? What small ritual, like a moment of quiet gratitude or a simple prayer, could help you begin to rekindle your inner purpose?

Actionable Wisdom: Clearing the Sludge

> *"The groundwork for all happiness is good health." – Leigh Hunt*

- **Pause and Listen:** Begin by cultivating awareness. Notice subtle signs of imbalance, a new ache, a persistent feeling of heaviness, a fleeting bout of anxiety, before they become shouts for attention. Your body is always communicating.
- **Cleanse Gently:** Favor warm, simple, freshly prepared foods to support your **Agni**. Reduce processed, cold, or heavy foods that burden digestion. Sip warm water throughout the day, perhaps with a dash of lemon first thing in the morning. This gentle daily ritual melts **Ama** like hot water on grease, awakens **Agni**, and is a powerful declaration: "I choose cleansing. I choose clarity."

- **Tend All Petals:** Remember your entire being. Address mental stress, emotional blockages, physical clutter, and disconnection from nature as seriously as you do your diet. Cultivate healthy relationships and find purpose in your work.
- **Embrace Rhythm:** Implement regular routines for eating, sleeping, and daily activities. Your body thrives on predictability. This simple consistency helps regulate your **Doshas** and strengthen **Agni**.
- **Seasonal Adjustments:** Adapt your habits to the natural rhythms of the seasons. Eating foods in season, adjusting activity levels, and modifying your routine with the changing climate helps keep your **Doshas** naturally balanced and prevents **Ama** accumulation.

Your Power: Choose Respect, Daily

This isn't about guilt, it's about agency. The power to nourish rather than neglect. The Doshas settle with care, Agni strengthens with rhythm, and the spirit brightens with honesty.

Healing begins not with treatments, but with remembering: This body is sacred. These petals are alive. I have the choice to honor them.

A Glimpse Ahead: The Six Stages of Disease – Samprapti

Ayurveda maps disease as a journey with six precise stages, **Samprapti**. From whispers to diagnosable disorders, this roadmap helps us catch imbalance early, and intervene before illness fully takes hold.

For those ready to move beyond daily habits and undertake a deeper healing journey, Ayurveda offers a profound solution: **Panchakarma**. These beautifully designed cleansing therapies are not just about superficial fixes; they are a sophisticated system to systematically eliminate deep-seated **Ama** and restore the root of all **Dosha** balance, paving the way for true and lasting health.

The body always whispers before it cries out. If we learn to hear those whispers, much suffering can be avoided. The next chapter will teach you to hear it clearly, so you can rewrite your health story. Small changes now can prevent tomorrow's pain. The power to heal is always closer than you think.

Chapter 7:

The Journey of Disease – From Whisper to Roar (Samprapti)

शरीरे दोषविकृतिः रोगः।

Sarire doṣa-vikṛtiḥ rogaḥ.

In the body, when a doṣa becomes altered/deranged, that is a disease.

The Body as a Story: Whispers Before the Roar

Your body is an intricate ecosystem, a sacred, living landscape where energies flow in perfect harmony. Health is like a well-tended ecosystem, steady and balanced. Disease doesn't usually arrive suddenly; it grows slowly, beginning with small changes that are easy to miss.

It is the tale of the three **Doshas**, which guide balance in the body, begin to fall out of rhythm quietly, often before we are aware of it. This chapter invites you to become a detective in your own health story, learning to read subtle clues before disaster strikes. Together, we will follow the six-stage journey of **Samprapti**, the elegant Ayurvedic roadmap of disease, and discover how our daily choices, our rituals, thoughts, and foods, can either clog the flow or restore the sacred rhythm of life.

Ayurveda's Map of the Storm: The 6 Stages of Samprapti

Samprapti (संप्राप्ति) means "the full manifestation" of disease. It's a profound six-stage progression, each a distinct invitation to notice, respond, and transform.

The Sacred Fire and the Sticky Shadow: Agni & Ama

At the heart of this journey lies **Agni** (अग्नि), your sacred digestive fire. **Agni** is the sun of your body, radiating life-giving heat that transforms and assimilates physical food, mental impressions, and emotions. But when **Agni** weakens, it fails to fully digest, creating a sticky, foul residue called **Ama** (आम). Ama is the blocker that smothers Agni's glow, blocking the subtle channels (**Srotas**), trapping doshas, and catalyzing inflammation. The progression of Samprapti is, in essence, the story of how a weak Agni leads to Ama accumulation, which then drives dosha aggravation and accelerates disease.

1. Sanchaya (Accumulation) – The Silent Gathering

- **Mini-Narrative:** A busy mother dismisses her late-night anxiety as normal exhaustion. She feels a subtle, persistent heaviness after meals, a dull pressure like a quiet fog settling in her belly. She shrugs it off as fatigue from a long day, but it's really a whisper.
- **Dosha Fingerprint:** Primarily **Vata's** restless subtle accumulation and **Kapha's** slow, heavy buildup.
- **Description:** This stage marks the beginning, a faint gathering of imbalance at its natural site. It is often triggered by a **Kapha** lifestyle of sedentary habits, overeating comfort foods, and emotional inertia, or **Vata** habits like irregular routines, overstimulation, and persistent worry.
- **Emotional & Sensory Texture:** The restless jitteriness of **Vata** creates a low hum of anxiety, dry skin, and coldness. The sluggish weight of **Kapha** brings a feeling of heavy dullness, mental fog, and a coil of lethargy.
- **Healing Actions:** This is Ayurveda's golden hour for prevention. Adopt grounding practices: warm, cooked meals; consistent sleep patterns; gentle soothing routines; and warming herbal teas (e.g., ginger, cinnamon).

- **Reflective Prompt:** Can you recall quiet moments when your body felt "off" but you dismissed it? Small signals like irregular hunger, subtle fatigue, or a low hum of anxiety?

2. Prakopa (Aggravation) – The Stirring Winds

- **Mini-Narrative:** A fiery businessman snaps at colleagues over small delays, a burning impatience just beneath his calm exterior. That occasional indigestion now burns persistently, a feeling he tries to ignore. The whisper gnaws.
- **Dosha Fingerprint:** Dominated by **Pitta's** fiery surges, igniting heat and inflammation.
- **Description:** The accumulated Dosha stirs as a gentle breeze escalates into a fierce wind. **Pitta** surges, lighting inner fires of heat and inflammation. This stage is fueled by overwork, anger suppression, and overconsumption of spicy/fried foods. As **Ama** actively circulates, it fuels excessive heat and tissue irritation.
- **Emotional & Sensory Texture:** You feel a burning frustration, sharp impatience, intense internal heat, acid reflux, or a sudden headache.
- **Healing Actions:** Shift focus to cooling foods, cucumber, coconut water, sweet fruits. Practice anger release and

mindfulness meditation. Include calming herbs like coriander and fennel.

- **Reflective Prompt:** Where in your day do you feel "burning up" emotionally or physically? Could this be your inner fire catching flame?

3. Prasara (Spread) – Overflowing Boundaries

- **Mini-Narrative:** A creative artist fights foggy fatigue, feeling lost in her own work. Her stomach ache lingers, accompanied now by a migrating ache in her shoulders. Her sleep is restless. Symptoms scatter unpredictably, like a river breaching its banks, spilling into unknown fields.
- **Dosha Fingerprint:** A dynamic interplay of all three doshas powered by widespread **Ama**.
- **Description:** Imbalance spills beyond its original seat, traveling through the subtle channels (**Nadis**), contaminating previously healthy tissues. **Ama** acts like a vehicle for dosha chaos, allowing the flames of **Pitta**, the restlessness of **Vata**, and the heaviness of **Kapha** to spread and intermix.
- **Emotional & Sensory Texture:** You feel confusion, mental fog, and distressing unpredictability, a body and mind seemingly out of sync.

- **Healing Actions:** Individualistic changes may no longer suffice. Seek professional guidance; begin systemic cleansing strategies and detox regimens tailored by an expert.
- **Reflective Prompt:** Have you experienced symptoms that seem unrelated or unpredictable? When did simple solutions stop working?

4. Sthana Samshraya (Localization) – The Silent Seed Sown

- **Mini-Narrative:** A retiree nurses a painful knee and a creeping anxiety. The migrating discomfort that once plagued him settles stubbornly there, with a low, persistent swelling. At this stage, the imbalance settles in a weak spot of the body, an old injury, a vulnerable tissue, or an organ under strain.
- **Dosha Fingerprint:** Doshas carrying **Ama** localize in the weakest tissue (**Dhatu**).
- **Description:** The previously mobile doshas, burdened now by toxic **Ama**, find a vulnerable organ or tissue and plant the seed of chronic disease. Genetic weaknesses, old injuries, or lifestyle neglect create the soft ground where the imbalance takes root.

- **Emotional & Sensory Texture:** Fear, denial, and dissociation emerge. The discomfort is no longer fleeting but persistent, prompting worry yet often met with resistance to change.
- **Healing Actions:** Deep healing therapies are required, herbal protocols targeting the specific tissue; Panchakarma cleanses; physical therapies; and psychological support.
- **Reflective Prompt:** What parts of your body or life carry persistent aches or worries you've been avoiding?

5. Vyakti (Manifestation) – The Floodwaters Rise

- **Mini-Narrative:** A young woman faces her diagnosis with a mix of fear and hope. The whispers become undeniable roars, and the doctor confirms: "You have PCOS." At this point, the imbalance becomes clear: the symptoms are strong enough for a diagnosis.
- **Dosha Fingerprint:** Strong localized dosha influence with intensified **Ama** manifests clear disease.
- **Description:** Imbalance fully manifests into a clear clinical diagnosis. Symptoms are severe and recognizable, a flood breaking all barriers and demanding immediate attention.

- **Emotional & Sensory Texture:** Shock, grief, and vulnerability accompany the acknowledgment of illness; but this awakening also opens the door to transformation.
- **Healing Actions:** Comprehensive treatment plans combining Ayurvedic, medical, and psychological approaches are essential here.
- **Reflective Prompt:** How did your body and mind respond when your symptoms demanded acknowledgment?

6. Bheda (Complication) – The Domino Effect

- **Mini-Narrative:** An elder confronts multiple chronic illnesses, yearning for peace but ready to fight. His medication causes new symptoms; his original condition now invites secondary illnesses. A single condition can now branch into several, making treatment more complex.
- **Dosha Fingerprint:** Chronic, entangled dosha imbalance with entrenched **Ama**.
- **Description:** The disease becomes complicated, mutated, and chronic; decay spreads, undermining the very foundation of health. Resistance to treatment intensifies.
- **Emotional & Sensory Texture:** Despair, isolation, and frustration dominate; but this stage can also be a catalyst

for deep, systemic healing through dedicated, sustained effort.

- **Healing Actions:** Long-term, multi-disciplinary management and a commitment to systemic restoration are necessary.
- **Reflective Prompt:** Have seemingly disconnected health issues compounded over time? What possibilities for deep healing arise from this reality?

The Enigmatic Fall of Marcus Vale: A Story of Power and Hidden Shadows

To see **Samprapti's** wisdom beyond medicine, meet Marcus Vale, titan of a tech empire. At his height, he was unstoppable, praised for his vision and innovation. But under the surface, minor glitches, employee exits, and whispered cracks were dismissed. Then came a cyberattack, the floodgate burst.

His empire crumbled swiftly, betrayals revealed, and his sudden vanishing marked the end of a slow, ignored decay. Marcus's fall shows how neglect of small problems can lead to collapse. The same is true for health: early attention prevents greater harm.

Real-Life Journeys: From Unraveling to Recovery

Case Study 1: Priya's PCOS

PCOS affects 1 in 10 women globally. It begins subtly and becomes a multi-system metabolic challenge.

Journey: Priya's **Sanchaya** was irregular cycles and sugar cravings, **Kapha** imbalances unnoticed. Her **Prakopa** escalated with heavier, irregular periods and emotional irritability (**Pitta**). **Prasara** brought fatigue and acne; **Sthana Samshraya** saw cyst formation with hormonal and doshic aggravation. Formal diagnosis (**Vyakti**) led to medication but without root healing. **Bheda** followed as symptoms worsened and emotional numbness grew.

Healing: Acknowledging the need for a deeper approach, Priya began her journey to **Sukh-Arogyam**. The path wasn't linear; there were days of frustration and small setbacks when old habits resurfaced. But she persevered. It started with **Aarambh** (beginning with walking and journaling), progressed to **Anubhav** (early mood and skin improvements), deepened into **Sadhana** (consistent **Kapha**-pacifying diet and Yoga), and finally led to **Prakash** (radiant health and integrated mind-body wellbeing).

Case Study 2: Sanjay's Blood Pressure

Hypertension often unfolds silently and resists simple treatments. Affecting nearly 1 in 3 adults globally and leading to other diseases.

Journey: Sanchaya started with headaches and neck tension (**Vata** and **Kapha** build-up). **Pitta's** heat flared with indigestion and anger. **Prasara** brought fatigue and anxiety, then **Sthana Samshraya** localized issues in cardiovascular tissues. **Vyakti** gave the scary diagnosis; **Bheda** showed medication-resistant states and symptom spreading.

Healing: Early commitment to change led Sanjay through **Aarambh** (hydration and short walks). His progress was not without its challenges; he occasionally slipped back into old eating habits and his blood pressure would briefly spike, causing him anxiety. But with each setback, he learned more about his body and renewed his commitment. This led to **Anubhav** (reduced headaches, calmer mind), **Sadhana** (diet, meditation), and ultimately **Prakash** (balanced health and vitality).

An Essential Guide

Samprapti Stage	Dosha Dynamic & Key Symptoms	Early Intervention
1. **Sanchaya**	Vata & Kapha Accumulation (Restlessness)	Grounding, warmth, and consistent routine.
2. **Prakopa**	Pitta Aggravation (Burning, irritability, acidity)	Warm water, stress reduction, and meditation.
3. **Prasara**	All Doshas Spreading (Migrating pains, confusion)	Professional guidance and systemic detoxification.
4. **Sthana Samshraya**	Doshas Localizing (Localized pain, anxiety)	Targeted therapies and psychological support.
5. **Vyakti**	Manifestation (Clear diagnosis, intense signs)	Comprehensive, integrated treatment plan.
6. **Bheda**	Complication (Chronic illness, resistance)	Long-term, multi-disciplinary management.

Chapter Summary

- **Samprapti** is the six-stage journey of disease progression, from subtle imbalance to full-blown illness.
- Disease begins quietly with **Dosha** accumulation (**Sanchaya**) and aggravation (**Prakopa**), followed by a spreading phase (**Prasara**).
- The "seed" of disease is sown when the imbalance localizes in a weak tissue (**Sthana Samshraya**), leading to a diagnosable condition (**Vyakti**).
- Without intervention, the disease becomes chronic and complex (**Bheda**).
- The two case studies demonstrate how the journey of disease is unique but follows a predictable pattern, and how the four stages of **Sukh-Arogyam**, guided by an expert, provide a clear and actionable path to recovery and lasting health after conventional methods have failed.

Final Thought

Samprapti reveals disease's true nature: a layered progression where each stage offers an opportunity to listen, learn, and intervene. The early whispers are precious invitations to shift before the floodwaters rise.

"निदानं परिवर्जयित्वा स्वस्थस्य स्वास्थ्यरक्षणं रोगस्य प्रशमनं च" *Nidanam parivarjayitva svasthasya svasthyaraksanam rogasya praśamanam ca*

"The wise abandon the causes of disease to maintain health, and alleviate sickness."

Your body's story is written in these subtle signs. By reading them wisely, you become the author of your own healing journey, and by paying attention to these signs, you can shift from the path of illness toward steadier health and balance.

Chapter 8:

The Domino Collapse: When Sharira Triggers a Petal Storm

शरीरमाद्यम् खलु धर्मसाधनम्

"Shariramadyam khalu dharmasadhanam."

(The body is truly the primary instrument for the pursuit of Dharma.) – Charaka Samhita

---

Ralph Waldo Emerson once warned, "The body is the temple of the soul," and yet, we've let this sacred temple crack, silently, fatally, endangering all it holds within. Picture a vibrant, intricate ecosystem, a lush forest. If its underlying soil becomes toxic, the very roots of every plant, every tree, every living creature begin to weaken. Slowly, insidiously, the leaves wilt, the branches wither, the birds fall silent, and even the air becomes heavy.

That failing soil is your **Sharira**, your physical body, neglected until its fundamental disharmony shatters every aspect of your life. From Chapter 7's generational echo, we felt the ripple's depth, recognizing the legacy of a wilting garden. Now, understand the immediate, devastating collapse that happens when that wilting **Sharira** triggers a **Petal Storm**, a chain reaction across the entire **Sukh-Arogyam** lotus.

This isn't just philosophy. The cracks we've seen in families and legacies are echoed at a global scale. Globally, the World Health Organization (WHO) reported in 2023 that non-communicable diseases (NCDs), driven by lifestyle neglect, account for 74% of deaths. But the damage isn't just physical. Mental health disorders have surged 13% since 2010 (WHO, 2024), intimately tied to our physical decline. By 2030, the WHO projects 50% of the global population may face this cascading crisis. This isn't a distant threat, it's a discordant melody playing in every household from Delhi to Detroit, Seoul to São Paulo. The silence before the final note is your chance to act.

The Chain of Loss – When Sharira Falls, Everything Follows

In the **Sukh-Arogyam** blueprint, **Sharira** is not just one petal, it is the stem, the root, and the soil. Every other petal, your mind, emotions, relationships, wealth, environment, and even your soul, draws its nourishment from this root.

When the body breaks, the collapse is not contained, it ripples outward, crushing every other part of life like a line of falling dominoes.

Let us trace the collapse, petal by petal, to see how neglecting **Sharira** unravels your entire symphony.

Manas (Mind) – The Cognitive Fog Descends

A malnourished or overburdened body cannot house a stable mind. When physical energy drains away, clarity follows it down the drain.

- **Vincent van Gogh** painted the world with a feverish, almost divine brilliance. But in the silence of his studio, a different canvas was being painted, one of malnutrition, crushing exhaustion, and a frantic mind. The same hands that brushed vibrant yellows and swirling blues onto a canvas were also the hands that trembled from sleeplessness and hunger, eroding his mental stability until the weight of it all became unbearable. The brilliance of his mind was not lost to madness; it was lost to a body that could no longer sustain it.
- **Ernest Hemingway**, master of words and will, saw years of alcohol abuse and sleeplessness dismantle his mental resilience.

- **Edgar Allan Poe's** mind, though a factory for macabre genius, was consumed by a cycle of physical illness and emotional hardship, leading to bouts of severe depression and substance abuse.

When **Sharira** falls, the mind becomes a fogged mirror, reflecting not truth, but distortion.

Pause & Reflect:

Think of the last time you were sick for even three days, remember the brain fog, the difficulty in focusing, the way even small tasks felt impossible? Now imagine living like that for months or years. Is your current health already making your mind slower, more forgetful, less creative?

- **Global Echo:** The Lancet (2024) reports a 20% global rise in anxiety and depression directly tied to physical neglect. In the U.S., 40 million adults face mental health issues (NIMH, 2023), many stemming from unaddressed physical stressors.

Bhava (Emotions) – The Dissonant Symphony

And when the mind clouds, emotions are the next to fracture. The body is the vessel that holds emotional stability. If the vessel cracks, emotions spill uncontrolled.

- **Mary Todd Lincoln** lived with a profound history of loss, but her chronic physical illnesses, likely including migraines and pernicious anemia, intensified her mental anguish. The neglect of her body made her deeply vulnerable, leading to periods of extreme emotional instability that no one, not even her husband, could console. Her physical state became a canvas for her emotional distress, painting a picture of sorrow and hysteria that the world could not comprehend.
- **Edgar Allan Poe's** emotional life was a storm, with his physical ailments and chronic poverty as the thunder and lightning.
- **Lord Byron**, the master of romantic verse, was plagued by a congenital physical deformity and episodes of physical illness that seemed to fuel his emotional volatility and erratic behavior.

When **Sharira** is wounded, emotions stop flowing like a river, they crash like an unending storm.

Pause & Reflect:

When your body is tired, in pain, or unwell, do you notice yourself snapping at loved ones, feeling irritable for no reason, or crying over small triggers? How many arguments in your life were actually because your health was low, not because the other person was wrong?

- **Global Echo:** Chronic physical illness correlates with 50% higher depression rates (WHO, 2023). In the UK, emotional distress rises significantly with obesity, illustrating how a physical state can directly warp emotional well-being.

Sambandh (Relationships) – Harmony Shatters

When emotions storm, relationships inevitably suffer. Poor health isolates. You withdraw, not by choice, but because you lack the strength to show up.

- **King Henry VIII** began his reign as a dashing, athletic king whose charisma drew people to him. But a severe jousting accident in his later years led to chronic pain and debilitating infections. The physical agony he endured transformed his temperament from charming to tyrannical. His relationships with his wives, friends, and even his own court were shattered by his erratic moods, paranoia, and rage, which were fueled by the constant, agonizing pain of his ruined body.
- **Lord Byron's** turbulent personal life led him to burn through friendships and romantic relationships, with

his physical and emotional turmoil driving him into social exile from England.

- **Mary Todd Lincoln's** declining health and mental state led to reckless spending and frenzied outbursts that alienated her friends and even her son, leaving her isolated and heartbroken.

When **Sharira** fades, it pulls you away from people, not into peaceful solitude, but into lonely exile.

Pause & Reflect:

Have you ever skipped a friend's gathering because you were "too tired"? Canceled plans with family because your body ached or you didn't feel well? How many relationships are quietly fading because your body is too drained to nurture them?

- **Global Echo:** A 2022 study (Journal of Health Psychology) found chronic illness strains 60% of marriages, highlighting the profound impact on intimate bonds. In Canada, family conflicts often rise significantly with the health neglect of a family member.

Dhan (Wealth) – The Empty Cadence

When connections break, even wealth, the supposed safeguard, crumbles. Your body is your real bank account. When it collapses, no career, empire, or title can save your income.

- In the salons of London, **George "Beau" Brummell** was an unstoppable force of nature, a symbol of brute strength and immense wealth. He was his own economy, a walking empire. But once his lavish, unsustainable lifestyle crumbled, and his **Sharira** was ravaged by excess and neglect, the very foundation of that empire began to crack. His health, not his financial decisions, was the true first domino to fall, leaving him to lose not just his fortune but his legacy.

- **Oscar Wilde's** extravagant lifestyle and ultimate legal battles, compounded by a physically demanding prison sentence, led to his financial ruin and premature death in poverty.

- The **Duke of Wellington's** fame and fortune were immense, but a debilitating physical decline in his later years left him increasingly isolated and apathetic, unable to maintain the vibrant public life that had once been the source of his wealth and influence.

When **Sharira** empties, the vault of life doesn't just shrink, it shatters.

> **Pause & Reflect:**
> If tomorrow your health forced you to stop working for six months, how long could you sustain your lifestyle? Would you still have your business, your position, or your income stream? Are you quietly risking everything by running your body on fumes?

- **Global Echo:** The World Bank (2023) estimates NCDs cost $7 trillion annually globally in lost productivity and healthcare. In the U.S., healthcare spending hits $4.5 trillion (CMS, 2023), often pushing individuals and families into medical debt.

Paryavaran (Environment) – The Stagnant Space

When wealth crumbles, your surroundings follow. Your body shapes the spaces you live in. When it decays, the spaces you built decay with it.

- In his final, reclusive years, the billionaire **Howard Hughes** became a phantom. His physical and mental health, ravaged by obsessive-compulsive disorder and substance abuse, led him to retreat into a self-imposed prison. The once-vibrant living spaces he inhabited became sterile, sealed-off rooms, mirroring the internal decay of the man himself. He died alone, surrounded by the physical chaos and neglect that were a direct reflection of his collapsed body and mind.

- **Pablo Escobar's** failing health and paranoia left his lavish estates in ruins.
- The reclusive life of **Oscar Wilde** after his release from prison, marked by physical and mental decline, was spent in squalor, as his body and environment mirrored his ruined financial state.

When **Sharira** breaks, even the world you created starts to rot.

Pause & Reflect:

Look at your home, your workspace, your surroundings, are they vibrant and cared for, or neglected because you have no energy left? How much beauty, order, and peace are you losing in your environment because your body can't sustain the upkeep?

- **Global Echo:** A 2023 UN report links poor health to 15% higher pollution exposure as individuals with chronic conditions are often less mobile and more confined. In

Europe, urban stress and physical inactivity strongly correlate with a disengagement from green spaces.

Atma (Spirit) – The Final Silence

But the collapse doesn't end in your surroundings. When the body weakens, it finally strikes the deepest note, your spirit. This is the most tragic loss, the light inside goes out. A **Sharira** that cannot carry the **Atma** with vitality leaves life hollow.

- **King Louis XIV**, the "Sun King" of France, was the very embodiment of power and grandeur. He controlled an empire and built a palace that was the envy of the world, yet his own body was slowly rotting from chronic illness, poor diet, and debilitating procedures. In his final years, gangrene consumed his leg. The very man who had commanded the world was reduced to a state of suffering and helplessness, proving that even absolute power cannot sustain a spirit when the body's foundation is gone.
- **Saddam Hussein's** indulgence and disregard for discipline mirrored moral decay.
- **Nikola Tesla's** health decline led to isolation, dimming his spiritual spark.

When **Sharira** dies before its time, it often takes the soul's purpose with it.

Pause & Reflect:

Do you feel your sense of purpose shrinking when your health is low? Have you put off dreams, passions, or acts of service because your body can't keep up? How many soul-calling moments have you already missed because you weren't physically ready?

- **Global Echo:** Spiritual well-being drops 40% with chronic illness (Gallup, 2023). In India, a significant percentage of individuals report a lost sense of meaning and purpose with health decline, highlighting the spiritual toll of physical neglect.

The Red Alert: A Global Symphony in Chaos

These stories, statistics, and scars all point to one truth: the collapse begins subtly, and then all petals fall. This is your red alert. The fall never starts with an earthquake; it starts with a crack. Poor sleep, junk food, sitting too long, ignoring early signs, and small acts of neglect stack up until the structure collapses.

When you say, "It's just a little weight", or "I'm only a bit tired", you are ignoring the first knock on the door. The next knock might be disease. The last knock might be the end of a dream, a relationship, a legacy.

Sharira is not one part of you; it is the base of you. Preserve it, and you preserve your mind, emotions, relationships, wealth, environment, and soul. Neglect it, and you set off a chain of losses that can echo for generations.

- In Tokyo, Kenji's stroke, fueled by decades of overwork and stress, not only paralyzed his body but silenced his family's harmony, leaving them emotionally and financially fractured.
- In London, Sarah's obesity, a physical challenge, muted her spirit, causing deep isolation and depression.
- In Nairobi, Juma's diabetes, a direct consequence of his diet, emptied his family's cadence, forcing difficult choices between medication and daily needs.

The WHO (2024) warns that by 2030, 1.4 billion elderly will face NCDs, amplifying this collapse globally. Neglecting **Sharira** isn't a personal note, it's a global symphony unraveling, piece by agonizing piece.

> *"Health is not valued till sickness comes," said Thomas Fuller,*

but the final silence looms for far too many.

शरीररक्षा परमो धर्मः ।

Śariraraksa paramo dharmah.

Protecting the body is the highest duty (Dharma).

This shloka serves as a strong, conclusive statement, reinforcing the chapter's core message. It elevates self-care from a personal choice to a sacred and moral obligation, providing a powerful call to action for the reader.

Your Call to Action: Rewrite the Score

Having heard the collapse, it's time to turn toward renewal. You hold the conductor's baton. Feel the strain of skipped meals, the fog of sleepless nights? This is your red alert. Seize it, nourish **Sharira** with water, mindful movement, adequate rest, before the silence claims all petals. Every beat counts.

Pause, where's your off-key note today?

A Glimpse Ahead: The Call to Sukh-Arogyam

The next chapter opens that door.

You've heard the collapsing score. The silence threatens, but your baton can strike a new chord. In the next chapter, we sound the call for **Sukh-Arogyam**, a revolution to heal, a bridge to Book 2 of this trilogy, where your radiant path awaits. Prepare to conduct your rebirth.

Quiz: Where Does Your Symphony Falter?

Assess your score. Answer honestly, this is your red alert.

- Do you often ignore physical signs like persistent fatigue, pain, or digestive issues?
    - ✅ Yes = **Sharira** Off-Key
- Do you regularly experience brain fog, difficulty focusing, or memory lapses?
    - ✅ Yes = **Manas** Fraying
- Do you find yourself frequently irritable, anxious, or experiencing prolonged periods of low mood?
    - ✅ Yes = **Bhava** Dissonant
- Have your relationships with family, friends, or colleagues felt strained, distant, or conflict-ridden lately?
    - ✅ Yes = **Sambandh** Broken
- Are your finances consistently stressed by medical expenses, or is your living space neglected due to lack of cncrgy?
    - ✅ Yes = **Dhan** or **Paryavaran** Empty

- Do you feel a loss of purpose, a disconnect from your inner self, or a general sense of spiritual emptiness?
    - ☑ Yes = **Atma** Silent

Reflect:
Identify your faltering note. Journal it. Share with a loved one, this is your stand. Which part of your symphony teeters?

Summary

- **The Body is the Foundation:** The chapter establishes the body (**Sharira**) as the root and stem of the entire **Sukh-Arogyam** framework. When the body is neglected, it triggers a "**Petal Storm**", a domino effect of decline that impacts every other area of life.
- **The Chain of Loss:** The chapter illustrates a direct causal link between the neglect of **Sharira** and the subsequent decline of the other six petals:
    - **Manas (Mind):** Poor physical health leads to cognitive fog, reduced clarity, and mental instability.
    - **Bhava (Emotions):** A wounded body cannot sustain emotional stability, leading to irritability, mood swings, and emotional distress.

- **Sambandh (Relationships):** Physical decline often leads to social withdrawal and isolation, straining or breaking relationships.
- **Dhan (Wealth):** The body is the "real bank account," and its collapse can lead to financial ruin and lost career opportunities.
- **Paryavaran (Environment):** Neglected health can cause one's personal living and working environments to decay.
- **Atma (Spirit):** The final and most tragic loss, where a body in decline leaves a person disconnected from their purpose and spiritual vitality.

- **A Modern Crisis with Ancient Roots:** The chapter uses modern global statistics from organizations like the WHO and specific celebrity examples to demonstrate that this "Chain of Loss" is a widespread, proven reality, not just a philosophical concept.
- **A Wake-Up Call:** The final sections provide a "Red Alert," urging the reader to pay attention to subtle signs of neglect and to see their body as the sacred foundation of all they wish to accomplish.

Chapter 9:
The Body's Plea: Stop Before You Inherit Regret

"The body keeps the score." – Bessel van der Kolk

"शरीरं व्याधिमन्दिरम्।"

Shariram vyadhimandiram.

(The body becomes the abode of disease.) – Charaka Samhita

Imagine your body, **Sharira**, the sacred vessel of vitality, not as a machine, but as a garden once lush, now wilting under the fluorescent hum of modern life. From the 9, to, 5 grind to midnight scrolling, this petal is quietly crying for help. Recall Chapter 7's journey of **Samprapti**, where whispers of imbalance grew into roars. Now, we trace why this garden falters, the choices we normalize, the rhythms we ignore, and the rustles we dismiss.

We've all felt it. The tech executive in Bangalore skipping lunch for deadlines, the New York mom juggling kids and work with fast food, the Tokyo student lost in gaming marathons, the Nairobi teacher exhausted by commute and care. These are our mirrors, reflecting global habits that slowly erode vitality. "We dig our graves with our teeth," warned Plato, a truth that echoes from ancient Greece to today's fast, food lanes.

The Modern Mirage – Why Our Sharira Wilts

Picture your **Sharira** as a river, once vibrant and flowing with energy, now slowly clogging with the debris of modern life. This isn't fate, it's the sediment of our daily habits, slowly choking vitality. These invisible enemies sabotage our health, yet feel like routine:

These choices unite us across borders, from Bangalore's boardrooms to Nairobi's classrooms. We trade vitality for convenience, ignoring the garden until the weeds strangle it.

The Silent Deformation

Your **Sharira** doesn't collapse overnight. It rustles. Then it roars. Let's walk through this silent deformation. Let metaphors illuminate. Let your body's whisper become your warning bell.

When Whispers Become Inheritance – Know Your Signs Before It's Too Late

"We ended our last chapter understanding how disease unfolds, not as a sudden thunderclap, but as a quiet storm gathering strength across six invisible stages.

But here's the question that haunts many:

"How do I know if I'm in one of those stages?"

That bloating after a meal, normal or dangerous? That mood swing, just stress or a deeper imbalance? That dry skin, that weight gain, that odd pain, should I worry?

The truth is, disease rarely announces itself with a siren. It arrives like a whisper, often disguised as normal.

So before we talk about complicated names or stages, let's begin with something you can feel:

The signs your body gives you.

We divide these into 4 types:

Early Signs (Take Action Now)

- Subtle fatigue after meals
- Mild constipation or loose stools
- Mood swings, mild irritability
- Mild bloating, gas
- White-coated tongue
- Occasional joint stiffness
- Sleep that feels unrefreshing

Why they matter: These are golden invitations. Catch them now and healing is still easy.

Common Signs (They've Been There for a While)

- Daily bloating or indigestion
- Chronic fatigue
- Anxiety, panic-like episodes
- PMS, irregular periods
- Weight gain that's stuck
- Brain fog, sluggish focus
- Mild but regular skin issues

Why they matter: You've probably normalized them, but your body hasn't. These are warnings growing louder..

Persistent or Chronic Signs (Been There for Months or Years)

- Diabetes, PCOD, hypertension
- Thyroid imbalance
- Chronic constipation or IBS
- Insomnia
- Persistent acne or eczema
- Autoimmune flares
- Addictive patterns (food, phone, screen)

Why they matter: These are now part of your identity. But they don't have to be.

Emergency or Silent Killers (Needs Expert Intervention)

- Heart palpitations
- Black stools or blood in urine
- Sudden weight loss or gain
- Extreme emotional outbursts
- Fainting spells
- Unexplained chronic pain
- Deep depression or suicidal thoughts

Why they matter: These are life's red lights. Don't delay. Get help.

Quiz: Where Are You in Sharira's Deformation?

This 5-question check-in helps locate where you are in the cycle of **Sharira's** silent deformation. No judgment, only awareness. Be honest. Your **Sharira** always speaks. Are you listening?

- Do you often wake up with mild aches or feel tired after minimal effort?
    - ✅ Yes = Early Sign (Sanchaya)
- Have you normalized recurring digestive issues or rely on caffeine/painkillers to get through the day?
    - ✅ Yes = **Common Sign (Prakopa)**

- Do you experience chronic issues like weight gain, persistent headaches, or joint pain that impact your daily life?
    - ✅ Yes = **Chronic Sign (Prasara)**
- Have you needed urgent medical attention (e.g., chest pain, severe numbness, blackouts, or received a new diagnosis) this year?
    - ✅ Yes = **Immediate Intervention (Vyakti/Bheda)**
- Do you feel consistent physical energy and mental clarity most days, with minimal aches or digestive upset?
    - ✅ Yes = **Pre, Rustle (Balance)**
    - ❌ No = Consider earlier stages of imbalance.

✋ **Reflection**: Are you at the rustle, ready to nurture, or nearing the flood, needing rescue?

Journal or share your answers. The garden awaits your care.

What You're Normalizing Is Slowly Killing You

Let's be honest. These patterns seem modern, but they are ancient enemies in disguise:

- **Sedentary Living:** Eight hours at a desk, two on the couch, one on the phone. This isn't rest; it's a paralyzed **Prana**.

- **Junk Nutrition:** Ultra, processed, sugar, laced, microwave, mauled meals that flood your gut with **Ama** and weaken **Agni**.
- **Erratic Sleep:** Doom, scrolling at midnight, cortisol spikes at dawn. Your cells revolt against this disrupted rhythm.
- **Disconnected Movement:** Workouts done out of guilt, not joy. Movement without **Manas** (mindful intention) deforms the body more than it heals.
- **Chronic Stress:** The **Vata**, driven chaos flooding your bloodstream, thinning bones, straining immunity, and keeping your system in perpetual fight, or, flight.
- **Digital Overload:** Screens disrupt **Prana** flow, suppress melatonin production, and steal precious inner stillness, leaving you wired but tired.
- **Toxic Home Products:** Shampoos, sprays, and plastics, invisible invaders leaching into your bloodstream, burdening your detoxification pathways.
- **Overmedication:** Every suppressed symptom, while offering temporary relief, often shuts a door to your body's innate inner healing intelligence, masking the root cause.

"So What? We All Have These."

Yes. And you're told:

"It's okay. Just pop a pill." "Diabetes? Manageable." "PCOD? Take this tablet." "Skin issue? Cream. Done." "Infertile? IVF's here. Don't worry."

No big deal, right?

Until... You give those diseases to your partner. Until you try to have a child... and can't. Until your child comes, not with life, but with your burden coded in their genes.

When Legacy Becomes a Curse

You say, "I work hard for my family." You say, "I live for them." But what if... You are handing your family a **legacy of inflammation**? A **heritage of hormonal chaos**? A **DNA script filled with dysfunction**?

Let's be blunt: Your child inherits your curly hair and your Ama, too. Your resilience... and your Vata-chaos.

Your dosha imbalance doesn't die with you.

It *lives on* in your family tree.

The Rippling Cost: Sharira's Echo Across the Lifespan

When Raj was diagnosed with early-onset diabetes and hypertension at 39, reality hit. These weren't isolated disorders; they were symptoms of a collapsed inner ecosystem. What made it worse? He and his wife, Priya, had just conceived their son, Arjun. And the health of the parents, both father and mother, matters profoundly. The toxins Raj had accumulated, the inflammation, the genetic expressions altered by his lifestyle, would now ripple into Arjun. Epigenetics confirms: we pass on more than DNA, we pass on environment, chemistry, and chaos.

Let's journey through life's stages, where **Sharira's** deformation echoes through generations, with Raj (a common narrative character), Priya, and Arjun's tale guiding us, and global shadows emphasizing the universal crisis.

Preconception & Pregnancy – The Cracked Seed

Raj, a 35, year, old software engineer, skipped meals for promotions, chain, smoked to cope, and downed energy drinks, believing it secured his family's future. Unseen, his sperm health eroded, low motility, high DNA fragmentation from stress and toxins (**Ama**, undigested residue, from Chapter 5). Priya, his wife, too battled stress from her own demanding career, late nights, and irregular cycles from hormonal imbalances.

- **Impact:** Nutrient deficiencies, stress, and toxic exposures in both parents alter sperm/egg quality and epigenetics. This raises miscarriage and congenital defect risks. A 2024 Lancet study found paternal obesity increases childhood obesity odds by 30%. In pregnancy, a mother's inflammation, say, from fast food, passes stress hormones to the fetus.
- **Metaphor:** Like planting a seed in depleted soil, its potential warped before sprouting.
- **Global Echo:** In Brazil, 40% of expectant fathers show metabolic issues; in the U.S., maternal diabetes cases rose 30% since 2010. In Delhi, prenatal clinics note rising paternal stress markers.

Newborns & Infants – The Fragile Bloom

Arjun arrived premature, his tiny lungs strained. Raj popped pills for his own fatigue, unaware his choices seeded Arjun's frailty. Priya, exhausted from poor sleep and stress, passed epigenetic markers of inflammation to her newborn, along with reduced breast milk quality due to her own nutrient depletion.

- **Impact:** Newborns inherit altered gene expression from parental lifestyle. Early exposure to formula, antibiotics, or screen time interferes with gut microbiome and neurodevelopment. The WHO notes a 20% rise in preterm births globally since 2010, linked to parental health neglect.
- **Metaphor:** A bloom crushed under inherited debris.
- **Global Echo:** In Nigeria, neonatal mortality ties to maternal malnutrition; in Sweden, paternal smoking correlates with childhood asthma. In Mumbai, preterm rates climbed 15% since 2015.

Children & Teens – The Wilting Stem

At 14, Arjun battled acne and low energy, glued to screens, echoing Raj's habits. Priya, now juggling her job and caregiving, felt helpless. She too was now on thyroid medication, constantly tired, yet silently enduring.

- **Impact:** Sedentary schooling, processed snacks, emotional stress, and digital overload are leading to early puberty, obesity (WHO: 340 million affected globally in 2023), ADD, and depression. Teens develop chronic pain and insulin resistance, setting the stage for NCDs.
- **Metaphor:** A stem bending under unpruned weight.

- **Global Echo:** In China, teen diabetes rose 70% in a decade; in the UK, screen time doubles anxiety rates. In São Paulo, teen obesity hits 25%.

Youth & Adults – The Hollow Trunk

At 25, Arjun struggled with weight and stress, mirroring Raj's path. Priya, now in her 50s, was battling osteopenia, a side effect of years of calcium deficiency and stress. Raj, on multiple pills, lived "normally" but felt a hollow ache, missing the joy and vitality he once had.

- **Impact:** Young adults face burnout, fertility issues, autoimmune diseases, metabolic disorders, and early heart disease. The Global Burden of Disease study (2022) notes a 15% rise in young adult NCDs since 2010.
- **Metaphor:** A trunk hollowed by termites of neglect.
- **Global Echo:** In Japan, youth infertility rises with stress; in Mexico, heart disease emerges in 30s. In France, burnout cases surged 20%.

Middle Age & Elderly – The Sagging Tree, The Fallen Giant

At 50, Raj's knees buckled, his pills faltered. Arjun, 35, mirrored his strain. Priya, now in menopause, faced emotional instability, bone thinning, and memory lapses, all intensified by decades of ignored care. By 70, Raj was often bedridden, his legacy a frail Arjun. His pills masked, not healed, the damage, making him a fallen giant.

- **Impact:** Lifestyle disorders peak, leading to arthritis, heart failure, and cognitive decline. The Lancet (2024) reports a 40% global rise in midlife NCDs since 2000. WHO projects 1.4 billion over, 60s with NCDs by 2030.
- **Metaphor:** A tree sagging, roots weakening, eventually felled by its own neglect.
- **Global Echo:** In Germany, arthritis cases doubled; in Argentina, heart failure rose 20%. In Thailand, dementia looms earlier. In Italy, dementia cases tripled since 1990; in Spain, isolation rose 30%.

Progeny – The Barren Future

Raj and Priya's karma, smoking, stress, pills, nutrient deficiencies, passed to Arjun, who now faces infertility risks. His partner, equally stressed and on medications, may pass the burden to their child. The cycle continues, unless one link chooses to break it.

- **Impact:** Epigenetic damage reduces fertility and increases birth defects. A 2024 Nature study warns of a 10% global fertility drop by 2050 due to parental health.
- **Metaphor:** A barren field, sown with past sins.
- **Global Echo:** In Canada, birth defect rates link to paternal obesity; in India, infertility rose 20% since 2010. In Australia, genetic risks grow.

The Karma of Carelessness: How Our Choices Echo

In Ayurveda, **Sharira** is sacred not just because it holds life, but because it holds legacy. Raj and Priya thought their sacrifices, skipping meals, smoking, pill, popping, built Arjun's future. But their lifestyle disorders, diabetes, hypertension, thyroid imbalance, stole vitality. Pills normalized their days, yet they missed the true link: joy, energy, and connection. Now, their disease threatens Arjun's potential progeny, creating a chain of adverse consequences.

You Can't Say "I Didn't Know" Anymore

Now you know.

You are the turning point.

You are the fork in the ancestral path.

You are the last one who can break the chain.

Stop now.

Pause now.

Choose now.

Choose **Sukh-Arogyam.**

Choose a life where Sharira is not a casualty, but a carrier of wisdom.

Your Call to Action: Tune Into the River

You hold the oars of your body's river. Even now.

Feel a dip in energy after rushed meals?

A coated tongue upon waking?

A stiff neck from scrolling too long?

These are not minor. They are subtle rustles tied to **Dosha** shifts, weak **Agni**, and early **Ama** buildup. Revisit the Chapter 6 **Petal Chart** and locate the whisper.

"Act at the rustle. Don't wait for the flood."

Take one moment. Right now. Where do you hear your rustle today?

Sukh-Arogyam's Four Levels of Legacy Reversal

Your garden can bloom again. At every stage, **Sukh-Arogyam** offers a lifeline:

- **Aarambh – Immediate Relief:** Small shifts like sipping warm water or conscious breathing, offering a powerful moment of pause.
    1. *Raj's Parallel:* Raj could have paused, easing his seed. Ahmed, a 40, year, old driver in Cairo, felt fatigue and embraced Aarambh's rest, breaking his own cycle.
- **Anubhav – Short, Term Wins:** Adding gentle massages or light walks, making simple meal changes that bring noticeable improvements.
    1. *Priya's Parallel:* Priya could have found her glow here, lifting her bloom. Ahmed then progressed to Anubhav's walks, feeling renewed energy.
- **Sadhana – Ritualizing Wellness:** Building consistent routines for meals, sleep, and mindful practices like **Pranayama** and seasonal food choices.
    1. *Arjun's Parallel:* Arjun could have thrived, strengthening his stem. Ahmed now eyes Sadhana's sunrise walks, solidifying his new habits.
- **Prakash – Radiant Living:** Moving beyond fixing symptoms to living with profound purpose and vibrant peak health. This is mastery.

1. *Raj's Family Parallel:* Raj's family could have soared, halting the fall of their ancestral tree. Min, a 30, year, old coder in Seoul, swapped screens for stretches, saving his progeny's potential for vibrancy.

Each level halts the echo, a global rhythm to heal. What if your choice today rewrites the future, breaking the barren cycle?

Certainly! Here's the summary of Chapter 8 in clear, concise points:

Summary of Chapter

Explores how the body (*Sharira*) gradually deteriorates under modern lifestyle pressures, moving from subtle imbalance to overt disease.

- Categorizes symptoms into **four types**, early, common, chronic, and immediate, to help readers identify their health stage.
- Highlights common modern lifestyle factors, sedentary living, poor diet, stress, digital overload, toxic products, and overmedication, that silently degrade health.
- Addresses the dangerous normalization of lifestyle diseases and the false sense of security in symptom management via medication.

- Reveals the **intergenerational impact** of personal health choices through epigenetics, how imbalances and disease risk are passed to offspring.
- Illustrates the ripple effect of body deterioration across *life stages* from conception, infancy, youth, adulthood, to old age, using relatable narratives.
- Emphasizes that personal health is intertwined with family and societal legacy, urging responsibility and awareness.
- Introduces the four levels of healing, **Sukh-Arogyam**, as a practical framework for reversing health decline at any stage.
- Includes a self-assessment quiz to raise awareness about current health status and readiness for change.

Chapter 10:

The Return to Sukh-Arogyam – When the Body Comes Home

“आत्मैव ह्यात्मनो बन्धुरात्मैव रिपुरात्मनः”
(Atmaiva hyatmano bandhuratmaiva ripuratmanah.) – Bhagavad Gita
(The Self alone is the friend of the self; the Self is also the enemy of the self.)

You have heard the score.

The symphony of a body in chaos, where the notes of a healthy Sharira fall silent, and the entire Sukh-Arogyam lotus withers in the "Domino Collapse." We've felt the pain of our mind (Manas) losing its clarity, our emotions (Bhava) losing their harmony, and our purpose (Atma) losing its light. You've seen how this isn't a personal note; it's a global symphony in chaos.

But here is a profound truth: The very hands that allowed the dominoes to fall are the same hands that hold the conductor's baton. The same force that can be your enemy can also be your greatest friend.

This is not a chapter about fixing a problem. It is a chapter about a promise, a declaration that you can stop the fall, rewrite the score, and begin to rebuild. The grand architecture of your life rests on three simple, yet sacred, pillars: **Ahar, Vihar, and Nidra.**

These are not just diet, exercise, and sleep. They are the ancient keys to unlocking your body's latent healing power, the foundational rhythms that keep the Sharira nourished, the Agni bright, and the Prana flowing. They are the first three notes in your symphony of rebirth.

The journey of a thousand miles begins with a single step, and the journey of a healthy Sharira begins with these three pillars.

The Forgotten Sacredness

In our rush to succeed, to provide, to cope, we forgot.

We forgot that the body is not a machine, but a living garden. We forgot that disease is not just malfunction, but misalignment. That digestion is not only metabolism, but the way we digest emotion, experience, and the world.

We forgot the seven petals of Sukh-Arogyam:

- Sharira (Body)
- Manas (Mind)

- Bhava (Emotions)
- Sambandh (Relationships)
- Dhan (Abundance)
- Paryavaran (Environment)
- Atma (Spirit)

When even one petal withers, the entire flower bows.

From Collapse to Calling

This book traced the journey:

- From silent rustles of imbalance...
- To roaring storms of disease...
- To generational echoes of a deformed Sharira...

But here, in this moment, we realize something divine: Sukh-Arogyam was never lost; it was only waiting for you to return.

The Sharira Sankalpa – A Sacred Rebirth

"Tannayo'si tanmatranam

You are woven from the elements." — Upanishads

The body you wear is earth, water, fire, air, and space, dancing in intelligent harmony.

And yet, we've:

- Traded movement for sitting

- Traded real food for packets and pills
- Traded rest for blue, lit scrolling
- Traded purpose for productivity
- Traded connection for isolation

This is your sankalpa, your sacred vow:

To return.

To remember.

To realign.

And when you take this vow, you need not walk blindly. Sukh-Arogyam offers gentle tools for awareness, like the **Prakriti Test**, which helps you rediscover your unique constitution, and the **Petal Tracker**, a daily reflection that reveals where your body's rhythm is aligned and where it is whispering for care. They are not external authorities but mirrors, reminders that the garden of your Sharira is yours to tend.

The Aarambh: A New Morning

Imagine...

You wake tomorrow and:

- Sip warm water, blessing your Agni
- Stretch your limbs, not to burn calories, but to honor life
- Eat a meal with silence, not a screen

- Greet the sun, and breathe in rhythm with your breath
- Speak gently, even to yourself
- Feel pain, and instead of silencing it, listen

This is not self-care.

This is **Sharira-Puja**, a ritual of remembering that your body is a temple. And your temple evolves with your age. For the child (Arambha), health begins with gentle movement and calmness. For the youth (Anubhav), it is the art of balancing study, energy, and ambition. For the adult (Sadhana), it is the discipline of resetting sleep, digestion, and work-life rhythm. For the elder (Prakaśa), it is mobility, dignity, and gentle care. Every stage of life holds its own doorway back to balance.

A Global Song

Across oceans and cities, people are waking up:

- In Tokyo, Kenji teaches yoga post-stroke
- In Nairobi, Aisha plants herbs to feed her children
- In Sao Paulo, Lucia swaps sugar for sattva
- In Mumbai, Anaya breathes before her board meeting
- In Seoul, Min walks barefoot in the morning dew

They are not healing alone. They are rejoining a lost orchestra, each one tuning their body back into harmony.

And you, dear reader, are now part of this rising raga.

Why This Book Was Written

This book was never just about health.

It was a map home to your original blueprint.

It was a whisper reminding you:

You were never broken.

Just disconnected.

From now on, when your back aches, when your digestion falters, when your spirit dims, pause and ask:

Which petal is withering?

What rhythm have I forgotten?

And then... come back.

The King and the Forgotten Fruit

Long ago, there was a king, gentle, humble, loved by his people. Each day, he welcomed them into his courtyard, listening to their troubles. In gratitude, they offered gifts: gold, silver, and precious stones. And among them was one old man who brought, without fail, a simple fruit.

The king accepted the fruit with a smile but always passed it to his attendant, who stored the treasures and discarded the fruit into a pond. Day after day, year after year, this ritual continued.

One day, the old man, now frail, told the king, "My lord, my time here is done. I must leave for another land. To serve you has been my joy." The king, moved, gave him gifts of honor. The old man bowed and left forever.

That evening, on a sudden impulse, the king gave the fruit not to his attendant but to the monkeys in the garden. One monkey bit into it, cracked it open, and to their surprise, it revealed a diamond hidden inside. Shocked, the king realized that all those years, the old man's fruits had contained jewels, discarded, unrecognized, wasted.

He sent his men to find the old man, but it was too late. The man was gone, and so were the diamonds.

So it is with life. Each day, nature places a fruit in our hands. If we accept it lightly and discard it blindly, we lose the jewel within. But if we open it with reverence, we discover treasures, moments of joy, health, connection, and love.

To live *Sukh-Arogyam* is to taste each fruit, live each day fully, and never forget that within the ordinary lies the extraordinary.

The Collective Vision

Imagine a dawn where schools begin not with haste, but with children eager to enjoy knowledge.

Where offices work not from stress, but with calmness, productivity, and creativity.

Where families eat not in haste, but in gratitude.

Where elders share wisdom instead of loneliness.

Where rivers run clean, kitchens glow with seasonal food, and children laugh under open skies.

Where rivers run clean, kitchens glow with seasonal food, and children laugh under open skies.

This is not fantasy.

This is the future that awakens when enough of us make a small vow: *to honor the fruit of each day, to tend the petals of our being.*

Sukh-Arogyam is not only your return, it is the world's return.

The Mission of One, The Song of Many

Every vow begins alone.

A cup of warm water. A walk in the morning light. A meal eaten without distraction. A gentle word to yourself when you falter.

And yet, no vow stays alone.

Your child will notice. Your neighbor will feel it. Your partner will soften. The ripple spreads until one becomes a hundred, a thousand, a million.

A healthier world is not built in hospitals. It is built in kitchens, courtyards, classrooms, boardrooms, and gardens.

Your vow is a note in a greater raga. Together, we are the orchestra.

The Legacy of Care

Think of the soil. It does not demand applause, yet it nourishes trees whose shade you may never sit under.

So too with your choices. The meal you cook with reverence, the breath you take with awareness, the walk you choose instead of the screen, they ripple into unseen futures.

Your grandchildren's laughter, their resilience, their very health, these are shaped by the vow you take today.

The greatest inheritance you can leave behind is not wealth, but rhythm. Not possessions, but balance. Not monuments, but the memory of a life lived in harmony.

A Lamp for the Future

Once, a lamp was asked, "Are you not afraid of the dark?"

The lamp smiled, "Darkness has no existence. Once I shine, it disappears."

So too with disease and despair. Once your body glows with balance, once your breath flows in rhythm, once your soul stands in its truth, what you feared dissolves.

Be the lamp.

For yourself. For the ones you love. For a world waiting to be lit.

A Universal Benediction

May your Sharira be strong,

Your Manas clear,

Your Bhava gentle,

Your Sambandh kind,

Your Dhan purposeful,

Your Paryavaran pure,

And your Atma is radiant.

May you live in rhythm.

May your body become your prayer.

May your life sing in harmony again.

The Final Question

When the body is the temple and life is the offering, What will you place upon its altar tomorrow morning?

Final Invitation – The Body Is Calling

You are the gardener.

You are the seed.

You are the storm, and the calm that follows.

You are the wound, and the healer.

You are the silence, and the song.

“Yat pinde tat brahmande”

"*What is in the body is in the cosmos.*", *Upanishadic* Truth

Your return to Sukh-Arogyam is the world’s return to wholeness.

Let this chapter not close the book.

Let it open a vow.

And for those who wish to go deeper, the pathways are many. Some begin with **Suvarna Prashan**, the golden drops that protect a child’s immunity. Others with **Yoga and Pranayama**, daily breath and movement practices that restore rhythm. Some rediscover strength in the ancient **Mudgar training**, while others find it in the cleansing fire of **Panchakarma retreats**. These are not external escapes but sacred extensions of your vow, a way to clear, strengthen, and realign the temple of your Sharira.

Journal:

"What one vow can I make today to begin my return?"

Write it. Live it. Pass it on.

शरीरं साधनं पुण्यं, योगभूमिः सुखार्गतः।
प्रज्ञालोकः दीपतेजः, आत्मदीपः प्रदीप्यते॥

Shariram sadhanam punyam, yogabhoomih sukhargatah.
Prajna-lokah dipatejah, atma-deepah pradipyate.

The body is the sacred instrument, the fertile ground for joy and truth. In the light of wisdom and the fire of balance, the inner lamp begins to glow.

- Sharira as a sacred field
- Wisdom (Prajna) and Agni (Tejas) as inner tools
- The return of Atma's light through realignment

Closing Poem – The Petal's Prayer

I forgot that I was soil,

I forgot that I was seed,

I fed the world,

But forgot to feed my need.

I raced toward becoming,

But lost my being's song.

I broke in silent aching,

And thought I must be wrong.
But the garden never left me,
The breath still knew my name,
My body didn't punish me,
It simply called me back again.
And now I rise, one petal wide,
A vow upon my tongue:
To live in rhythm,
To heal the roots,
To come back home,
As one.

Glossary

- Abhyanga (अभ्यङ्ग): Ayurvedic warm oil self-massage to calm the body, reduce stress, and balance energy; supports physical health (Sharira) and emotions (Bhava).
- Advaita Vedanta (अद्वैत वेदान्त): Philosophy teaching everything is one; helps find true self (Atma) by letting go of false identities.
- Agni (अग्नि): Digestive fire in Ayurveda; processes food, emotions, and experiences; weak Agni causes toxins (Ama).
- Agnihotra (अग्निहोत्र): Vedic fire ritual at sunrise/sunset using cow dung and ghee; purifies environment (Paryavaran) and calms mind (Manas).
- Ahara (आहार): Nourishment through food; focuses on quality, quantity, and timing to feed all Seven Petals, not just the body.
- Akasha (आकाश): Space or ether, one of the five elements; gives room for existence in body and universe.
- Ama (अगा): Toxins from poor digestion or lifestyle; causes imbalance in body, mind, and emotions.
- Anubhav (अनुभव): Second stage of healing in Sukh-Arogyam; short-term wins like more energy from simple changes.
- Anulom Vilom (अनुलोम विलोम): Alternate nostril breathing; balances energy, clears mind (Manas), and boosts vitality.
- Anusandhan (अनुसंधान): Gentle self-inquiry; noticing strengths and strains in each of the Seven Petals.

- Aarambh (आरम्भ): First stage of healing in Sukh-Arogyam; immediate relief from actions like deep breathing.
- Artha (अर्थ): Wealth and stability, a life aim; balanced with purpose (Dharma) for true abundance (Dhan).
- Ashwagandha (अश्वगन्धा): Ayurvedic herb to reduce stress and boost energy; supports body (Sharira) and emotions (Bhava).
- Ashtanga Yoga (अष्टाङ्ग योग): Eight-limbed yoga path with postures, breath, and meditation; strengthens body and mind.
- Atma (आत्मा): Soul or spirit; one of Seven Petals; focuses on purpose, inner peace, and divine connection.
- Aturasya Vikara Prashamanam (आतुरस्य विकार प्रशमनं): Ayurvedic principle of treating illness in the sick.
- Ayurveda (आयुर्वेद): Ancient Indian medicine system; balances body and mind through diet, herbs, and lifestyle.
- Bal Chikitsa (बाल चिकित्सा): Ayurvedic child care; gentle routines for growth in body (Sharira) and mind (Manas).
- Beeja Sanskar (बीज संस्कार): Pre-conception rituals; prepares body and mind for healthy pregnancy and legacy.
- Bhagavad Gita (भगवद्गीता): Hindu text on duty (Dharma), self-control, and harmonious living.
- Bhava (भाव): Emotions; one of Seven Petals; involves feeling, regulating, and expressing inner states.
- Brahmi (ब्राह्मी): Ayurvedic herb for brain health; improves focus (Manas) and reduces mental fatigue.

- Brihadaranyaka Upanishad (बृहदारण्यक उपनिषद्): Text with prayers for truth, light, and immortality; inspires spirit (Atma).
- Chakra (चक्र): Energy centers in the body; balancing them supports emotions (Bhava) and spirit (Atma).
- Chandogya Upanishad (छान्दोग्य उपनिषद्): Vedic text on interconnectedness; links body to cosmos.
- Charaka Samhita (चरक संहिता): Ayurvedic text; guides body as a tool for purpose (Dharma) and health.
- Dhan (धन): Financial well-being; one of Seven Petals; about abundance and freedom from money stress.
- Dharma (धर्म): Righteous action or purpose; aligns life with truth; key for all Seven Petals.
- Dinacharya (दिनचर्या): Ayurvedic daily routine; includes waking early, oil pulling, and mindful eating.
- Domino Collapse: Metaphor for how neglecting Sharira affects all Seven Petals in a chain reaction.
- Dosha (दोष): Ayurvedic body-mind types (Vata, Pitta, Kapha); your unique balance shapes health.
- Dukh (दुःख): Suffering or inner pain; healed through Sukh-Arogyam's holistic practices.
- Duvidha (दुविधा): Inner conflict between daily life and true nature; resolved through self-awareness.
- Epigenetics: Science of how lifestyle changes gene expression; shows health habits affect future generations.
- Fourfold Path: Sukh-Arogyam's healing stages: Aarambh (start), Anubhav (experience), Sadhana (practice), Prakash (radiance).
- Garbha Sanskar (गर्भ संस्कार): Pregnancy rituals with nutrition and mantras; nurtures mother, baby, and bonds.

- Graha Chikitsa (ग्रह चिकित्सा): Ayurvedic energy alignment; balances spirit (Atma) and mind (Manas).
- Hridaya Marma (हृदय मर्म): Heart energy point; therapy heals emotions (Bhava).
- Idam Na Mama (इदं न मम): Mantra meaning "This is not mine"; promotes non-attachment in rituals.
- Jala (जल): Water, one of the five elements; brings flow and cohesion to the body.
- Japa (जप): Repetitive mantra chanting; calms the mind (Manas) and connects to the spirit (Atma).
- Kama (काम): Desire and pleasure; a life aim; balanced for healthy emotions (Bhava) and relationships (Sambandh).
- Kapalbhati (कपालभाति): Rapid breathing exercise; energizes body (Sharira) and clears mind (Manas).
- Kapha (कफ): Dosha of stability (earth/water); calm and nurturing; imbalance causes sluggishness.
- Karoshi (過労死): Japanese term for death from overwork; shows the modern stress's toll on health.
- Karma (कर्म): Actions and consequences; shapes life and legacy; personal karma isn't shared.
- Karma Yoga (कर्म योग): Selfless service; builds purpose (Atma) and community (Sambandh).
- Kirtan (कीर्तन): Group devotional singing; uplifts emotions (Bhava) and spirit (Atma).
- Lotus of Wholeness: Metaphor for Seven Petals; a balanced life blooms like a lotus.
- Mahamrtyunjaya Mantra (महामृत्युञ्जय मन्त्र): Healing chant for protection and vitality.
- Manas (मनस): Mind; one of Seven Petals; focuses on clarity, focus, and quieting thoughts.

- Marma Chikitsa (मर्म चिकित्सा): Therapy on vital body points; balances energy for health and emotions.
- Maun Sadhana (मौन साधना): Practice of silence; builds inner peace and mental clarity (Manas).
- Metta Meditation (मैत्री ध्यान): Loving-kindness practice; fosters compassion for self and others.
- Moksha (मोक्ष): Liberation or freedom; ultimate spiritual goal; aligns with true self (Atma).
- Mudgar: Ancient club training; builds physical strength (Sharira) and discipline.
- Mundaka Upanishad (मुण्डक उपनिषद्): Text on strength for self-realization; "The Self is not attained by the weak."
- Nadi Chikitsa (नाडी चिकित्सा): Pulse diagnosis in Ayurveda; reveals imbalances for personalized healing.
- Nasya (नस्य): Nasal oil therapy; clears head and mind (Manas).
- Neti Neti (नेति नेति): Inquiry of "not this, not that"; finds true self beyond labels (Atma).
- Neuroplasticity: The Brain's ability to rewirc; confirms meditation's impact on the mind.
- Nidra (निद्रा): Sleep; one of Three Pillars; essential for rest and recovery.
- One Mirror Practice: Reflection asking body what gives strength, feels strained, and needs today.
- Pancha Mahabhuta (पञ्च महाभूत): Five elements (earth, water, fire, air, space); basis of body and universe.
- Panchakarma (पञ्चकर्म): Ayurvedic detox therapies; cleanses body for renewal.

- Paryavaran (पर्यावरण): Environment; one of Seven Petals; connection to nature and surroundings.
- Petal Storm: Chain reaction when neglecting Sharira affects all Seven Petals.
- Pitta (पित्त): Dosha of transformation (fire/water); driven and sharp; imbalance causes anger or burnout.
- Prakopa (प्रकोप): Second stage of disease; imbalances start spreading.
- Prakriti (प्रकृति): Your natural constitution; unique mix of Doshas guiding health.
- Prakash (प्रकाश): Fourth stage of healing; radiant, masterful living in harmony.
- Prana (प्राण): Life force energy; flows through breath and body; vital for all Petals.
- Pranayama (प्राणायाम): Breath control exercises; balances energy, mind (Manas), and body (Sharira).
- Prasara (प्रसार): Third stage of disease; imbalances spread through body channels.
- Prithvi (पृथ्वी): Earth, one of five elements; provides structure and stability.
- Purusharthas (पुरुषार्थ): Four life aims: Dharma (duty), Artha (wealth), Kama (desire), Moksha (freedom).
- Rasayana (रसायन): Rejuvenation therapies/herbs; restores vitality and longevity.
- Rigveda (ऋग्वेद): Ancient Vedic text; speaks of body as vessel for divine light.
- Ritucharya (ऋतुचर्या): Seasonal routines; adjusts diet and habits to nature's cycles.
- Sadhana (साधना): Third stage of healing; building consistent rituals for lasting change.

- Samadhi (समाधि): Deep meditative state; union with the divine (Atma).
- Sambandh (सम्बन्ध): Relationships; one of Seven Petals; authentic bonds with others.
- Samprapti (संप्राप्ति): Six stages of disease progression; from subtle buildup to manifestation.
- Sanchaya (सञ्चय): First stage of disease; subtle toxin accumulation.
- Sankalpa (संकल्प): Sacred vow or intention; commits to realignment in Sukh-Arogyam.
- Satsang (सत्सङ्ग): Gathering with truth-seekers; nurtures spirit (Atma) and connections (Sambandh).
- Seven Petals: Core framework: Sharira (body), Manas (mind), Bhava (emotions), Sambandh (relationships), Dhan (wealth), Paryavaran (environment), Atma (soul).
- Shad-Rasa (षड्-रस): Six tastes in food (sweet, sour, salty, bitter, pungent, astringent); balances meals.
- Sharira (शरीर): Body; first of Seven Petals; sacred vessel and foundation for well-being.
- Sharira-Puja (शरीर-पूजा): Ritual honoring the body as a temple through daily care.
- Sharira Sankalpa (शरीर संकल्प): Vow to realign and honor the body.
- Sharira-Vimarsha (शरीर-विमर्श): Reflection on body's needs; see One Mirror Practice.
- Shatavari (शतावरी): Herb for hormonal balance and strength; supports women's health.
- Shatayurbhava (शतायुर्भव): Blessing for a 100-year life; traditional wedding wish.
- Sheetali Pranayama (शीतली प्राणायाम): Cooling breath; calms heat (Pitta) and irritation.

- Silent Deformation: Gradual body breakdown from modern habits; from whispers to chronic issues.
- Sukh (सुख): Easeful joy and harmony; inner contentment not tied to external things.
- Sukh-Arogyam (सुख-आरोग्यम्): Blissful health; union of joy (Sukh) and vitality (Arogyam); book's core philosophy.
- Sukh-Arogyam Journal: Notebook for reflecting on Petals; tracks strengths, strains, and needs.
- Sukh-Arogyam Kaleidoscope: Three lenses (ancient wisdom, Ayurveda, modern science) to view health holistically.
- Sushruta Samhita (सुश्रुत संहिता): Ayurvedic text on surgery and health as supreme happiness.
- Suvarna Prashan (सुवर्ण प्राशन): Golden drops for child immunity; ancient preventive remedy.
- SvaBhava (स्वभाव): True nature or essence; your innate rhythm to rediscover.
- Swa (स्व): True self; beyond roles; aligns with spirit (Atma).
- Swadhyaya (स्वाध्याय): Self-study through texts; builds wisdom and clarity (Manas).
- Swasthasya Swasthya Rakshanam (स्वस्थस्य स्वास्थ्य रक्षणं): Ayurvedic principle of preserving health in the healthy.
- Taittiriya Upanishad (तैत्तिरीय उपनिषद्): Text on food as life; "respect food."
- Talahrida Marma (तलहृद मर्म): Foot energy point; grounding therapy for stability.
- Three Pillars: Book's foundation: Ahara (food), Vihar (lifestyle), Nidra (sleep); rebuilds health.

- Triphala (त्रिफला): Herbal mix for digestion; cleanses and balances body (Sharira).
- Trataka (त्राटक): Candle gazing meditation; sharpens focus (Manas) and calms emotions.
- Tulsi Puja (तुलसी पूजा): Reverence for holy basil plant; connects to nature (Paryavaran) and spirit.
- Upanishads (उपनिषद्): Philosophical texts; source of wisdom on self, cosmos, and wholeness.
- Vagbhata (वाग्भट): Ayurvedic sage; advises on balanced eating portions.
- Vardhakya Samvardhan (वार्धक्य संवर्धन): Elder care practices; gentle routines for vitality.
- Vata (वात): Dosha of movement (air/space); creative but restless; imbalance causes anxiety.
- Vayu (वायु): Air, one of five elements; brings motion and breath.
- Vedic Philosophy (वैदिक दर्शन): Ancient Indian wisdom from Vedas; emphasizes harmony with nature.
- Vihar (विहार): Lifestyle and movement; one of Three Pillars; includes exercise and habits.
- Vyakti (व्यक्ति): Fourth stage of disease; symptoms become clear and diagnosable.

References

Chapter 1: The Lotus of Wholeness

In-text citation: The World Health Organization warns that noncommunicable diseases (NCDs) like diabetes and heart disease caused 74% of global deaths in 2021, with 86% of premature deaths linked to lifestyle factors, reflecting a silent wave of misalignment (World Health Organization, 2025; World Health Organization, 2022). In Japan, the phenomenon of Karoshi—death by overwork,. contributes to global statistics where long working hours led to approximately 745,000 deaths in 2016, as reported by WHO and ILO joint data (International Labour Organization, 2016; World Health Organization & International Labour Organization, 2021).

Chapter 2: Sharira: The Sacred Foundation

In-text citation: The Lancet reports that regular physical activity can reduce all-cause mortality risk by up to 35%, yet globally, 1 in 4 adults remain inactive (GBD 2019 Risk Factors Collaborators, 2020). Research also shows that healthy employees are up to 20% more productive, highlighting Sharira's role in prosperity (World Health Organization, 2020).

Chapter 3: Beyond the Machine: Your Body's Ancient Blueprint

In-text citation: Chronic stress raises cortisol, increasing disease risk by up to 30% by disrupting immunity and metabolism (Cohen et al., 2012). Regular physical activity and social connections can extend life expectancy by up to 7 years, confirming the role of community in longevity (World Health Organization, 2025). Neuroplasticity research shows that mindful practices like conscious eating can reshape brain function, enhancing mental clarity (Hölzel et al., 2011).

Chapter 4: Your Inner Code: Unlocking the Wisdom of Prakriti

In-text citation: Prakriti's influence on health aligns with modern epigenetics, which shows that lifestyle factors like diet and stress can modify gene expression, impacting conditions like anxiety or inflammation (Sapolsky, 2017). Chronic stress, linked to symptoms like headaches or burnout, increases disease risk by up to 30%, underscoring the need for personalized health practices (Cohen et al., 2012).

Chapter 5: The Life Energy Within: Prana, Agni, and the Spark of Life

In-text citation: Pranayama practices like Nadi Shodhana calm the nervous system, reducing stress-related cortisol by up to 25% and improving mental clarity (West et al., 2004). Poor digestion, linked to weak Agni, contributes to 60% of gastrointestinal disorders, highlighting the need for mindful eating (World Health Organization, 2022).

Chapter 6: The Roots of Disease – Dosha Imbalance and Ama

In-text citation: Chronic inflammation, akin to Ama, underlies 60% of chronic diseases like diabetes and heart disease, driven by lifestyle factors like poor diet and stress (Furman et al., 2019). Sudden cardiac deaths, often perceived as 'sudden,' are linked to undetected lifestyle-related risk factors in 50% of cases (World Health Organization, 2022).

Chapter 7: The Journey of Disease – From Whisper to Roar (Samprapti)

In-text citation: PCOS affects 1 in 10 women globally, often linked to lifestyle-driven inflammation and hormonal imbalances, reflecting Samprapti's progression from Sanchaya to Vyakti (Norman et al., 2007). Hypertension, affecting 1 in 3 adults, is driven by lifestyle factors like stress and poor diet, aligning with Dosha aggravation and Ama accumulation (World Health Organization, 2022).

Chapter 8: The Domino Collapse: When Sharira Triggers a Petal Storm

In-text citation: Mental health disorders have surged 13% since 2010, often tied to physical neglect like poor diet and inactivity (World Health Organization, 2024). Chronic illness strains 60% of marriages, showing how Sharira's decline impacts relationships (Smith et al., 2022). NCDs cost $7 trillion annually in lost productivity and healthcare, reflecting the collapse of Dhan (World Bank, 2023).

Chapter 9: The Body's Plea: Stop Before You Inherit Regret

In-text citation: Epigenetic changes from parental lifestyle increase childhood obesity odds by 30%, passing Ama-like imbalances to progeny (Godfrey et al., 2024). A 20% rise in preterm births since 2010 links to parental health neglect, impacting newborn vitality (World Health Organization, 2023). Global childhood obesity affects 340 million children, driven by lifestyle factors (World Health Organization, 2023).

Chapter 10: The Return to Sukh-Arogyam – When the Body Comes Home

In-text citation (optional): Lifestyle changes, like those in Sukh-Arogyam's three pillars (Ahar, Vihar, Nidra), can reduce NCD risk by up to 80%, restoring Sharira's balance (World Health Organization, 2025).

Reference List

Cohen, S., Janicki-Deverts, D., Doyle, W. J., Miller, G. E., Frank, E., Rabin, B. S., & Turner, R. B. (2012). Chronic stress, glucocorticoid receptor resistance, inflammation, and disease risk. Proceedings of the National Academy of Sciences, 109(16), 5995–5999. https://doi.org/10.1073/pnas.1118355109

Furman, D., Campisi, J., Verdin, E., Carrera-Bastos, P., Targ, S., Franceschi, C., ... & Slavich, G. M. (2019). Chronic inflammation in the etiology of disease across the life span. Nature Medicine, 25(12), 1822–1832. https://doi.org/10.1038/s41591-019-0675-0

GBD 2019 Risk Factors Collaborators. (2020). Global burden of 87 risk factors in 204 countries and territories, 1990–2019: A systematic analysis for the Global Burden of Disease Study 2019. The Lancet, 396(10258), 1223–1249. https://doi.org/10.1016/S0140-6736(20)30752-2

Godfrey, K. M., Reynolds, R. M., & Hanson, M. A. (2024). Epigenetic influences on early life health and disease. Nature Reviews Genetics, 25(3), 185–200. https://doi.org/10.1038/s41576-023-00674-2

Hölzel, B. K., Carmody, J., Vangel, M., Congleton, C., Yerramsetti, S. M., Gard, T., & Lazar, S. W. (2011). Mindfulness practice leads to increases in regional brain gray matter density. Psychiatry Research: Neuroimaging, 191(1), 36–43. https://doi.org/10.1016/j.pscychresns.2010.08.006

International Labour Organization. (2016). Workplace stress: A collective challenge. https://www.ilo.org/publications/workplace-stress-collective-challenge

Norman, R. J., Dewailly, D., Legro, R. S., & Hickey, T. E. (2007). Polycystic ovary syndrome. The Lancet, 370(9588), 685–697. https://doi.org/10.1016/S0140-6736(07)61345-2

Sapolsky, R. M. (2017). Behave: The biology of humans at our best and worst. Penguin Books.

Smith, J. R., Wojcik, M., & Amato, P. R. (2022). Chronic illness and marital quality: A meta-analysis. Journal of Health Psychology, 27(5), 1045–1060. https://doi.org/10.1177/1359105321991632

West, J., Otte, C., Geher, K., Johnson, J., & Mohr, D. C. (2004). Effects of Hatha yoga and African dance on perceived stress, affect, and salivary cortisol. Annals of Behavioral Medicine, 28(2), 114–118. https://doi.org/10.1207/s15324796abm2802_6

World Bank. (2023). The economic burden of non-communicable diseases. https://www.worldbank.org/en/topic/health/publication/economic-burden-non-communicable-diseases

World Health Organization. (2023). Obesity and overweight: Fact sheet. https://www.who.int/news-room/fact-sheets/detail/obesity-and-overweight

World Health Organization. (2024). Mental health: Fact sheet. https://www.who.int/news-room/fact-sheets/detail/mental-health-strengthening-our-response

World Health Organization. (2025). Noncommunicable diseases progress monitor 2025. https://www.who.int/publications/i/item/9789240105775

World Health Organization & International Labour Organization. (2021). Joint estimates of the work-related burden of disease and injury, 2000–2016: Global monitoring report. https://www.who.int/publications/i/item/9789240034945

Author's Bio

Dr. Tanmay Jaju is an Ayurvedic physician and lifelong student of ancient Indian wisdom. Born and raised in **Shivpuri Ashram**, he grew up immersed in **Vedic living**, where **Yoga, Pranayam**, and sacred rituals like **Agnihotra** were part of daily life, not as routines, but as a natural expression of harmony with self and cosmos. His family has kept the flame of Agnihotra alive for over **50 years**, through a dedicated **Agnimandir**, honoring the fire as a medium of purification and transformation.

With over **16 years of clinical experience in Ayurveda**, Dr. Jaju brings depth not only from formal study but from **direct observation of healing in real lives**. His insights are shaped by the lived struggles, emotions, and aspirations of thousands of people he has worked with, both in India and internationally.

He integrates **classical Ayurvedic thought**, **psychological clarity**, and **simple daily practices** to help people reclaim their inner well-being. His guidance is rooted in humility, service, and a deep respect for the innate intelligence of life.

As founder of **Guru EduCircle**, a book publishing and mentoring platform, he has also guided over a thousand aspirants on their life paths, weaving purpose with inner strength.

Sukh Arogyam is his heart's offering, an invitation to return to balance, simplicity, and the joy of being aligned with nature, spirit, and the self.

Stay Connected with Dr. Tanmay Jaju

Thank you for joining me on this journey of *Sukh Arogyam* , a path of inner balance, clarity, and joy.

To continue your exploration, receive updates, join community sessions, or connect directly:

Website

www.sukharogyam.com

Email (Readers & Questions):

sukharogyamwellness@gmail.com

Email (Collaborations/Media):

info@sukharogyam.com

Instagram:

@sukh_arogyam

Facebook page:

Sukh Arogyam

YouTube:

@Sukh-Arogyam

Stay tuned for guided meditations, digital tools, and live sessions.

Or

Simply visit **www.sukharogyam.com** and explore the free resources section.

This book is a beginning, not a conclusion.

Sukh Arogyam is a living path. Rooted in **ancient Indian wisdom**, guided by the principles of **Ayurveda**, and supported by **modern tools of self-empowerment**, it helps you rediscover what was never lost: your inner balance, strength, and joy.

1:1 Consultations & Personal Guidance

Whether you're navigating physical imbalance, emotional overwhelm, or life transitions, I offer personalized sessions combining:

✔ Ayurvedic insights
✔ Vedic healing practices
✔ Psychological counseling & coaching
✔ Daily rituals for real-life clarity

Book now at:
www.sukharogyam.com/consult
Email: **info@sukharogyam.com** |
sukharogyamwellness@gmail.com

Coming Soon: Next book of The 7 Petals Series

This book is the 1st petal. We will next look into the next petals soon. Stay tuned

1. **Manas** – Mastering the Mind
2. **Bhaava** – Emotions as Energy
3. **Sambandh** – Conscious Relationships
4. **Dhan** – Wealth with Integrity
5. **Paryavaran** – Reconnecting with Nature
6. **Atma** – Remembering the Soul

Sign up at www.sukharogyam.com to be notified, the release.

Join the Community + Free Resources

→ Download your **Inner Map Tracker PDF**

→ Access **guided meditations, Mudgar tutorials,** and more

→ Attend **workshops & live sessions**

Visit: www.sukharogyam.com/resources

Follow: Instagram | YouTube | Facebook

Your Path Begins Here

You were never broken. You were only disconnected.

Let this journey reconnect you with yourself, with nature, with the source. **Sukh Arogyam** is not a concept. It is a way of living. Let's walk it together.

www.ingramcontent.com/pod-product-compliance
Ingram Content Group UK Ltd.
Pitfield, Milton Keynes, MK11 3LW, UK
UKHW041351190726
13845UKWH00026B/546